## Commendations for *Facing Cancer: Standing Together*

"It can be easy to feel you are just a number, especially in the health service. Adrian and Karen completely dispel any notion that you are not an individual or that you are unimportant in God's eyes. They tell how God has spoken to them, individually and repeatedly, through his word as they submit to the circumstances he arranges for them. An encouraging and challenging read."

**Lloyd Gilpin,** *local GP*

"This book—*Facing Cancer: Standing Together*—reminds me of some words by Elizabeth Prentiss (1818–78 and author of the hymn, 'More Love to Thee, O Christ'):

> *The thorny path bears some of the sweetest flowers that adorn life; and when with naked, bleeding feet we walk upon a flinty soil, we often find diamonds. But nobody believes that, save those who have dared the thorn and the flint, plucked the flower and seized the gem.*

Adrian and Karen's captivating and heart-tugging story is certainly one of having 'dared', 'plucked' and 'seized' together. In the Lord's providence, he has wonderfully made and matched them for this journey, all for his own glory and honour."

**Pamela Gaiya,** *Mission Africa Field Facilitator, Nigeria*

"What has kept Adrian and Karen Adger so cheerfully serving others in the face of incurable cancer? Read their story and you will discover this secret: they are ***together*** standing tall. By being open with each other and their community they get strength to face every day together—together as a couple, together with their wider family and friends, together with the church, together with caring professionals, together with print/music and video partners, and, above all, together on their knees before the Lord Jesus. Trouble and tragedy can often distance us from God and even lead to division in families and communities. Karen and Adrian show us a better way."

**Rev Dr Sid Garland,** *International Director-at-large, Africa Christian Textbooks (ACTS)*

"I first got to know Adrian Adger in the late 1980s when we served the Lord together doing Youth Fellowship work in our local churches in Ahoghill, County Antrim. I have always known and been inspired by Adrian as a humble and zealous follower of Jesus Christ. In this book, *Facing Cancer: Standing Together,* Adrian and Karen talk honestly about his battle with cancer. This book is God-centred and gospel-centred. It will both move you and fill you with Christian hope. At a moment when there is much uncertainty and fear, surely this is a book for such a time as this. It is a privilege to endorse it and I do so with a whole heart."

**Rev Stephen Johnston,** *minister, Kilkeel Presbyterian Church*

"I first met Adrian Adger in 1991 when we were full time students at Belfast Bible College. Almost immediately we struck up an amazing friendship and twenty-nine years on Adrian is still my best friend. Adrian always longed to find a godly wife and I prayed with him about this special request. They say good things are worth waiting for and that came in the form of Karen Anderson. I had the joy and privilege of conducting their wedding on 23 July 2013. Karen has been an amazing support to Adrian and, as you read this book, there is no doubt that as they faced cancer they have stood together! I warmly commend this book to you."

**Rev Brian Smyth,** *minister, Trinity Presbyterian Church, Ahoghill*

"It is a privilege to recommend this book to you. I met Adrian over thirty years ago—back then, Adrian had a passion for the gospel and a desire to reach out with the message of saving grace which has only intensified over the years. And Karen has such a kind and loving heart for people and a great love for the Lord and his work. We were thrilled when the Lord brought them together and have seen the hand of the God in every aspect of their lives and ministry. God has blessed them in many ways and, even through these dark days of illness, the Lord has proved his ever-present help and strength to them as they face cancer, standing together. Adrian' s first book, *Facing Cancer: Standing Tall* has helped, encouraged and strengthened many who are going through similar circumstances and we know that this book will also be a blessing to people right across the world."

**Keith Lindsay,** *Acre Gospel Mission*

"*Facing Cancer: Standing Together* captivated my attention and thrilled my soul right to the end of the book. Here is a couple living with the shadow of death over their lives 24/7. Sunshine and clouds, highs and lows, mountains and valleys—they are all here. Adrian and Karen bare their souls and tell it like it really is. Yet shining through this 'dark providence', we see a couple who adore the Lord, appreciate his pardon, adore his person, acknowledge his people, accept his providence and anticipate his prospect. Yes, all these themes are here. Read it for yourself—and, like Adrian and Karen, you will be able to say, 'Through it all, through it all, I've learned to depend upon his Word.'"

**Denis Lyle,** *retired Baptist pastor*

# Facing Cancer: Standing Together

*A Christian couple's story of finding peace*

by Adrian and Karen Adger

Published by Adrian and Karen Adger

Contact:
Clough Presbyterian Church
18 The Square, Clough, Downpatrick, County Down BT30 8RB

Seaforde Presbyterian Church
Demense Road, Seaforde, Downpatrick, County Down BT30 8SG

www.cloughandseaforde.com

Print bookISBN 9781999327064
e-book ISBN: 9781999327071

First edition 2020



Printed and bound in the UK

# Contents

# Foreword

It is my immense privilege to write the Foreword to this wonderful new book by Adrian and Karen Adger.

I have known Adrian for quite a few years now. He impressed me very positively—right from the time of our first meeting—as a man of profound Christian maturity and spiritual depth. As we have fellowshipped together over the years, first in overseas mission with Mission Africa and then in ordained ministry in the Presbyterian Church of Ireland, this man of God has always been a huge encouragement and blessing to me. Humble and self-effacing, Adrian lives out the Christian faith with vivid reality and tenacity. You too will be blessed as you read here his wise insights and observations.

Adrian has been blessed immeasurably in life by his lovely wife Karen, and readers will be moved and uplifted by her testimony of their life together. It is a joy to read of God's gracious dealings in her life. Just as in life, so as in writing, they are a formidable team and together are an encouragement and inspiration to the people of God.

You should expect to be challenged in this book. The contents are not simply a series of comforting feel-good anecdotes. Rather, this is a story of real life in its rawness, a story that does not shy away from dealing with physical, mental and spiritual pain. But those qualities alone do not summarise the power of this book. It poses the most significant of questions—what will you do with the claims of Christ on your life in the most extraordinarily challenging circumstances? Here, we read Adrian and Karen's glorious Christ-centred response to that question. For this is not a book in which Adrian and Karen promote themselves—they point the reader to the Lord Jesus.

I end by giving thanks to God, for having led Adrian and Karen to write this book.

*Rev Dr W J Paul Bailie,*
*CEO, Mission Africa, July 2020*

## Chapter 1

# Finding out

'It will just be a routine scan.' That's what one person had said to us. In April 2017, a cancerous tumour had been found in my kidney—and both the kidney and the tumour had been removed. All the lymph nodes around the kidney were clear—so, after the operation, we were informed that no further treatment was necessary. Fast forward to Monday 6 November 2017: the date of my six-monthly scan. Karen and I travelled by car to Craigavon Area Hospital in County Armagh to receive the results.

The consultant's words were stark and clear: 'Now this is really out of the blue.' We weren't expecting this. That wasn't good. There were new lesions in my abdomen and they were inoperable and incurable. It was an unbelievable shock. He said he was sorry he could not have done more. We thanked him for what he had done.

### Why us?

We travelled home trying to digest the news. We were in a state of shock—completely disorientated and so confused. Trying to understand it all seemed way beyond us and we had so many questions. Why? Why me? Why now? Why this? It felt so unfair. We wept all night. We were overwhelmed and devastated. It was like our worst nightmare actually happening. We kept asking each other, is this really happening?

I had only recently married Karen, and I didn't want to leave her. I had recently become the minister in Clough and Seaforde Presbyterian churches. I didn't want to leave this calling. We felt a tremendous sense of loss. Our hopes and dreams had gone up in smoke. We just couldn't believe what had happened. We couldn't take it in. I was only fifty-four years old and I felt I was being cut down in the midst of life. It felt like an immediate death sentence.

How can I describe that time? We were constantly in tears. It was disturbing and unsettling. Real pain and stress. It was like a dark cloud coming over my life. I wondered if I would would ever know joy again in my life. Was I finished?

## Last sermon?

At a funeral service I was conducting on Boxing Day 2017, I was talking to two men (not from our congregations) who said that they heard that this would be my last sermon and that I was resigning as a minister at the end of December. I said that was not the case. Yet I wondered if I had long left to live, let alone work.

Karen and I took a week's holiday at the beginning of January 2018 because we thought this could be our last holiday together. Chemotherapy would also begin later in January and I wanted to keep working, although one of the cancer nurses said that it was was unusual for anyone to be working while on chemotherapy. We faced a great deal of uncertainty. We knew we had no control over our future. Does anyone have any control over their future? Was the result of the next scan simply like tossing a coin? Heads, it's a good result; tails, it's a bad result. Was it simply an accident that we received such a bleak cancer diagnosis? A stroke of bad luck? Would good luck or bad luck lie ahead? Should we simply 'touch wood, all will be well'? Maybe we needed more faith, if we had enough faith then everything would work out? Maybe what we needed was some positive thinking? Some people say that if you have a positive outlook, then you will recover, whereas negative thinking brings you down.

Since then, like all those who are faced with a serious cancer diagnosis, we have had multiple hospital appointments—scans, scan results and treatment. And, on top of that, in recent months, the

Covid-19 pandemic has emerged as a threat to the whole world and to all of our lifestyles.

Where do we turn when our lives have been turned upside down and we have no answers? Where do we turn when we feel we have no future and we are in a dark place? Where do we turn when difficulties seem to be overwhelming?

Such difficulties seem to threaten our faith. John Piper said this: 'There is no weapon like the Word of God for warding off threats to faith.'[1] As we turned to God's precious Word, the Bible, we found great comfort and reassurance. In the changing circumstances of life, we were able to turn to the unchangeable Scriptures of the Old and New Testaments. Personally, I have also received tremendous love and support from my wife Karen, as well as friends, family and the church family. We have been overwhelmed by the encouragement we have received from so many people and from a wide spectrum of evangelical churches.

Of course, my bleak cancer diagnosis affects Karen's life most of all. Karen is my wife, whom I love dearly, she is my soulmate and my main carer. Karen has been a tremendous support to me. How is she personally coping with it all? Sometimes the carer is forgotten about and ignored, as the focus is on the person who is ill—yet the carer carries the heaviest burden of all. Let Karen tell her story.

*She swallowed a fly,*
*Perhaps she'll die...*

For some reason, we always seemed to sing this particular song as dad took us for a walk down the Ballybrick Road. My sisters and I would join hands and skip in a row from one side of the road to another. On one warm May afternoon, I was on a school trip and our group had just finished our picnic lunch. I began coughing and coughing, aware that something was stuck in my throat. There was only one thing going through my eight year old mind, I must have swallowed a fly, just like the old woman, and we all know what happened to her!

I was extremely anxious to get home to mum, my tummy was doing somersaults, and I was gripped with a growing fear. Something else was taking priority—my immortality. I knew from an early age that I needed to be saved. My godly parents took me to Rathfriland Baptist where I was taught in Sunday school every Sunday afternoon and so I knew the gospel story. That afternoon, I was face-to-face with death and, for the first time, hell was a real place and I was afraid to go there. I got home that afternoon but, instead of explaining my plight, I kept it secret. Instead, I kept going to the bathroom to try to cough up the fly.

## Bedtime traumas

Bedtime came round and it must have been late, as my parents were also up to bed too. I was in and out bed like a yo-yo, convinced that time was running out, and that the fly would strike me dead at any moment. I was going to die. I could stick it no longer. I crept along the short stretch of landing to my parents' room which was ajar. My dad was asleep and so I silently tapped him on the arm and whispered, 'Daddy, I want to get saved. Daddy, I want to get saved now.'

Despite the fact that I had just woken him out of sleep, he didn't hesitate, but lifted his large Bible that was sitting on the bedside cabinet and we proceeded back to my bedroom that I shared with Lynne. I got back into bed and my dad knelt by the bedside turning the Bible pages to the book of Romans. He read to me from chapter 10, verse 9.

> *If you openly declare that Jesus is Lord and believe in your heart that God raised him from the dead, you will be saved.*
> (New Living Translation)

He took his time carefully explaining the way of salvation to me and I prayed verse 9 as a sinner's prayer, trusting that if I declared Jesus was Lord and if I believed in my heart that God raised him from the dead, then I would be saved. I laid my head on my pillow after that prayer. All fear now gone, sins now forgiven, now on my way to heaven with no more worry about going to hell.

## Assurance

However, I still had a problem, I had a fly in my throat and so I thought to myself, 'One last attempt, Karen. You can do this!' That was my final trip the bathroom sink that night. One almighty cough and up it came. I looked at it in the palm of my hand, lifeless. It wasn't a fly at all! To my absolute amazement, it was just a tiny, insignificant, little apple pip. That little apple pip had been lodged in my throat for around ten hours, perfectly intact until that precise moment. Coincidence? I believe I had to accept God's offer of mercy through faith and trust in him before the apple pip was uncovered. The Bible makes it very clear in 2 Corinthians 6:2 that today is the day of salvation, now is the time of God's favour.

His favour was upon me as an eight year old child and I received it. What about you, dear reader? Nothing in this life is guaranteed, only right now. I was sharing my new faith the next day in primary school, telling everyone they needed to be saved. I was so excited and amazed at what the Lord Jesus had done for me.

I said at the beginning that I had a wonderful childhood, and we made our own fun together as siblings and as a family. Beside us lived our wonderful grandparents whom we saw every day, although sadly I lost my beloved Nanna in my later teens. As children, we went every Tuesday evening to the gospel bus which was a children's meeting in the Friends Hall in Rathfriland. We were picked up by the bus at our home by 'Uncle Sammy' as he was affectionately known. We also had Sunday school every Sunday afternoon at 3 o'clock in the church—and we were also prone to having our own 'church' at home on the living room floor, with dolls on the cushions! My brother David did the preaching. No television on Sundays was the norm in our home as children.

As I reached the age of eleven or twelve, I was old enough to go to youth fellowship. The youth fellowship leaders in the church were Leonard and Margaret Graham and I absolutely adored them from the start, especially Margaret. They loved us as young people and it was so evident by their commitment and interest in each and every one of us. As I reached the age of fifteen, our pastor—the late Edward Rea—was taking the youth fellowship. As a group, we were at a stage of really wanting to learn. I still recall this godly man talking to us about subjects like justification, sanctification and others, and expounding the Word of God to us. When I think back now, I remember the amazing times we had with Pastor Rea, then also with Pastor Keith Lindsay. Both Keith and his wife Karen are still good friends of ours. They took the youth fellowship in their home on Sunday evenings after Keith had already preached at services that day. Before I was married I was enjoying the ministry of the current Pastor of the church, Ian Wilson. The church has continued to flourish under his excellent leadership. Adrian and I always receive a warm welcome and we have much appreciated their continued prayers and support.

I am so humbled by the sacrifice they made for me and so many others. Now, being married to a minister, I am able to understand and appreciate the physical stamina and the spiritual strength needed to do that. That is what real love for the Lord Jesus and his sheep, including the lambs in the flock, is all about. They were investing in us and I know that I am the person I am today because of my youth leaders and pastors. Their love, concern and interest in me spiritually is still bearing fruit in my life today. If you are a Sunday school teacher or youth leader, your calling to teach the young is not simply a box-ticking exercise. Children and youth may not always appreciate your efforts, but you are sowing a seed that will bear fruit in God's time. It is easy to become discouraged as we serve, especially if we see little or no fruit for our effort at the time. We are encouraged in Galatians 6:9 to not be weary in doing good, for in due season we shall reap a harvest if we do not give up. And in Psalm 27:14, 'Wait on the Lord, be strong and take heart and wait on the Lord.'

## Hospitality

I was a student in Rathfriland High School and, throughout school, I was in the same class as Pastor Jonathan Rea (Pastor Edward Rea's son). I didn't enjoy school and looked forward to leaving. I had a summer job in a guest house in Newcastle and it was here that I discovered my love for hospitality. I knew that I would like to attend Banbridge Technical College after High School, to study Catering and Hospitality. My two years in Banbridge were two very enjoyable years. I had wonderful opportunities here to speak about my love for the Lord Jesus.

I absolutely loved my course and I got a job in a restaurant in Banbridge after completing it. I was confident this was my start on the career ladder to an executive chef position. I was never an overly competitive person but I took absolute pride in my work and it had to be the best. Things changed, however, when my employers bought their own premises in the town of Bangor which is on the coast, an hour away by car from my home. I was offered a new job if I decided to go with them. I was nineteen years old, with my whole life ahead of me. I accepted the offer as my other option was unemployment! I didn't know if I was a home bird or not—but I was about to find out very quickly. I remember mum leaving me at my new room in the home of an elderly lady and the floodgates opened widely. I was miserable from day one—but I was prepared to give it a go.

A few weeks into my new life in Bangor, I wasn't any happier and what began was a dedicated search to discover God's will for my future. This was a major turning point in how I viewed prayer and in my personal reliance on the Lord. Prayer for me was on my knees begging the Lord to intervene in my circumstances. It was also specific targeted prayer regarding a new job. I gave my life completely in service to the Lord and was willing to go wherever he wanted me to go.

## Life at the Castle

At that time, a new young couple had taken over management of Castlewellan Castle Christian Conference Centre in Castlewellan, a twenty-minute drive from my home town of Banbridge. They were settling in and it wasn't long before they were seeking a new cook. What happened next was amazing. God was at work behind the scenes directing all things for my good. I received a phone call from my mum asking me if I was interested in a job there. How amazing is God! A new job, just twenty minutes from home—but, more importantly, I was exactly in the centre of God's will for my life.

I ended up having almost nineteen years of happy, rewarding ministry serving in the Castle. It was during my time in the Castle that the Lord brought into my life my best friend, Sarah. We have been through thick and thin together. I have so many memories that I could share but a really special one was when I got married to Adrian. Sarah stayed with me the night before the wedding. We did a last-minute visit to the venue and the next day, my big day, she was there to take me to the hairdresser and then help me into my dress. In May 2017, I had the joy of watching her get married. The day was tinged with sadness as Adrian was recovering from his kidney operation and therefore couldn't attend. And, not only was he not with me, he had to forego the great privilege of conducting the service due to his illness. However, God was gracious and my dad was able to step in and bring a message to the newly-weds—the Lord always goes far beyond our expectations and he is able to do immeasurably and abundantly more than we can ask or think (Ephesians 3:20). Sarah and I are sisters in the Lord, as she knows Jesus personally for herself. Added to that, her husband Trevor is my sister's brother-in-law! So one big happy extended family.

I cannot talk about the Castle without saying a little more about my previous boss, Andrew Forson, and his wife, Lorna. Andrew and Lorna began managing the Castle three months before I joined the team. Andrew was a wonderful boss, and very kind, and they served so well together. God is using them both in wonderful ways in Castlewellan Castle and it was my privilege to be part of that 'family'. I was so blessed and privileged to be working for a Christian charity. It is a wonderful blessing for Northern Ireland to have such a place. Many have been encouraged, strengthened and nurtured in their faith in Christ, all because they have been to Castlewellan. Pray for Castlewellan Castle and other Christian conference centres and retreats in our province, that God will continue to bless them as they take their stand for Christ.

I had to learn quickly on my feet as I was previously working in a restaurant, and the type of catering in the Castle was on a different level completely. I still remember my first weekend and a group of thirty people were coming to stay for the weekend. Thirty people was daunting. Fast forward a few weeks and I was preparing and serving meals for one hundred plus people. I had a real love and passion for my work and to serve the church in this way was so fulfilling for me. We had a variety of groups who came to stay—from church family groups, youth clubs, youth fellowships, girls and boys brigades, and missionary groups, to name a few.

## Embracing diversity

My eyes were opened to the diversity in the evangelical church and it was a learning experience. I was able to see that not everyone does church the same way—and that's fine! I was learning much back then and the Lord was preparing me for my future as the wife of a Presbyterian minister. There are many Christians who say they love to stay in the background and they are not upfront in ministry. Yet they do play a vital role in the body of Christ, as all members of his body are crucial. I would have classed myself like that as I worked and served in the ministry in the Castle, and I do believe it is a vital ministry serving the family of God.

## Grateful guests

I loved it when someone came at the end of the weekend or the week and just said 'thank you'. I received many cards and gifts over the years from grateful people. I remember one occasion when Andrew came to me and shared that there were a few young men staying during the week and to expect to see them around, but that they were going to be fending for themselves. Men fend for themselves—yeah, right! I felt sorry for them and so I left food and desserts up in their lounge area during their stay, and had opportunity to chat to them. I didn't see them leave but they kindly left me chocolates, flowers and a scribbled note signed… Rend Collective. They were in the early days and what an amazing band they have become, with a global singing ministry. Another remarkable guest was the late Dr Helen Roseveare, a missionary with Worldwide Evangelization Crusade, who was speaking at a missionary conference. Andrew and Lorna did whatever they could to help everyone and they continue to bless others in the Castle today.

I loved my years working in the Castle and can say that the Lord really blessed me in that time and I made lifelong friends. How sweet it is to be in the Lord's will for your life. We are all on a mission as believers. We don't all have to be called to deepest Africa, and we won't be—so, therefore, our mission is in our everyday employment, our home life, and out and about in our local community. That's our frontline, where we can be most effective in service for Jesus Christ.

## Chapter 3

# Finding a man

In March 2012, I met Adrian Adger. I was working away in the Castle—but my life was about to move in a completely different direction.

I remember Andrew once sharing with me that being unhappy does not mean that we are out of God's will. I never forgot that. So often as Christians, when things go wrong, we can jump to the rash conclusion that we must have slipped out of God's will. We are told in Philippians 4:11 to be content with whatever we have and in Colossians 3:22-24 we are to obey our earthly masters in everything, to please them all the time, not just when they are watching you. We are to serve them sincerely because of our reverent fear of the Lord. We are to work willingly at whatever we do, as though working for the Lord rather than people. Verse 24 concludes by saying, 'since you know that you will receive an inheritance from the Lord as a reward. It is the Lord Christ you are serving.'

### Settled and single

I knew that I was in God's will for my life but he was about to change things. Both Adrian and I knew ourselves that we didn't want to consider dating if the relationship may not seriously go somewhere. I was thirty-eight years old and very settled in my life. There can be a misconception, even in Christian circles, that you have to be married in order to be settled and happy. This is not correct, in my humble opinion. I do believe singleness is a real struggle and even a burden for many and it can be hard to accept that the Bible does view singleness as a gift. I was very aware when I gave my life to the Lord, to serve him fully, that there would be sacrifice on my part. I believed that my position at the Castle was best suited to that of a single person. There was a lot of weekend work, including Sundays and early mornings, and those of you who are in catering know it can be very unsociable.

Before meeting Adrian, I remember chatting on the phone with my friend James (who also happened to be a friend of Adrian's, and would later be our best man). I asked him what his plans were for Saturday night. His reply—'I am meeting my friend, Adrian'—to which I replied, 'Who is Adrian?' I didn't know who this Adrian was and why was he not in our circle of friends who 'ran about together'. As I probed further to satisfy my own nosiness, I was hit with 'Adrian's a great fella but not the man for you'...!

James shared how Adrian was studying for the Presbyterian ministry. As I was a 'dyed in the wool' Baptist, the conclusion was that we would not be suited. So that was my introduction to Adrian Adger. About eight months later, in March 2012, I met Adrian in the flesh. That evening, I was with another really good friend, Millicent, and was meeting others for dinner in the village of Broughshane, just outside Ballymena. I really believe that God brings good friends into our lives through many different ways. Milly, as she is affectionately known, and I had both been going through painful situations in our lives and the Lord helped us through those times together. I think of the verse in Proverbs 17:17, 'A friend loves at all times', and Milly comes to mind, as she's a loyal friend. It is important as Christians to have good friends, including unbelievers, as we need to be close to people in order to reach them for the Lord. At the same time, I strongly believe our godly Christian friends are the ones whom we should seek in times when we need help and wise counsel. I particularly love the New Living Translation of Proverbs 27:9, 'The heartfelt counsel of a friend is as sweet as perfume and incense.'

So, Milly and I were almost the last to arrive that evening at the restaurant and I sat down at the table—not realising that my future husband was just a few chairs away. We enjoyed the craic (or good fun, for those who need a translation!) and we left, still completely unaware of Adrian's footsteps behind us as he walked along with our friend, Roger. Later that evening, after a Christian meeting, the moment in time had come when God had planned for us to speak! I was standing outside and spied a friend chatting to a very tall man. Now for any of you ladies reading this who are over 5 ft 10, you will know that tall Northern Ireland men are a bit of a novelty! I shimmied over and blurted out, 'You know my friend James.' I had his attention immediately. There was a brief conversation which I can't recall now but I know I made an impression.

## Chance encounters?

That was the beginning of a string of 'meetings'. Milly and I were then invited to a barbecue and guess who was there? That evening, I knew Adrian was interested and, sure enough, the next day our mutual friend James rang me to see if I would meet Adrian for a coffee. I thought about it and my head went straight to 'but he's a Presbyterian'—and, worse than that, was training to be a Presbyterian minister. I knew we would have a few doctrinal differences and, on that basis, I couldn't consider his gesture of meeting for a coffee.

A week later, Milly and I were at a Christian meeting and across a crowded tent, I saw Adrian. I spoke to him afterwards—I think I had a guilty conscience from the previous episode. The conversation was so natural and flowing and I know the Lord was playing match maker. The next day, I asked James to send me Adrian's number. We arranged that afternoon to meet up for dinner the following Thursday. Did I buy a new dress for our first date? Of course I did! I had all kinds of thoughts swirling through my head as I got ready that evening, mainly denominational ones. I received lots of encouragement from my friends Alan, Karen and Belinda in the Castle, and Andrew and Lorna were behind me too.

When I arrived in the little carpark across from the Indian restaurant in Newcastle, Adrian was parking in the same place. Feeling confident in my new dress, I ordered my favourite Indian dish! The conversation flowed but I had those typical first-date nerves and I couldn't finish my meal. Being on my home turf, we headed afterwards to the promenade and walked towards the Slieve Donard Hotel. We ordered our coffee which we shared on a cosy settee—not too cosy—and chatted until we were told that they were closing. I was ready to call it a night, but Adrian was keen to stay a bit longer. He also wanted to meet up soon after, but I was hesitant and put the brakes on. I knew though that I had met someone really amazing—but I was still debating our doctrinal differences in my mind.

## Good company

The Lord was definitely working and I found that every time I saw Adrian, his spirituality was more and more attractive. I deeply believe that Christian character is of upmost importance in our relationships and that we are defined by our character. In Romans 5:3-5 we read:

> *Not only that, but we rejoice in our sufferings, knowing that suffering produces endurance, and endurance produces character, and character produces hope, and hope does not put us to shame, because God's love has been poured into our hearts through the Holy Spirit who has been given to us.* (English Standard Version)

In contrast we read that bad company corrupts good character (1 Corinthians 15:33). Therefore, it's imperative that we seek a godly partner with godly character. I believe this includes our closest friends and allies. Adrian and I were now seeing each other regularly and we officially became an item at the end of June. The summer time was always busy at the Castle, as groups stayed from Saturday to Saturday, and Adrian was on summer break from his studies at Union Theological College. Andrew was so kind by allowing

Adrian to stay over on occasions at the Castle over those summer months. It really gave us an opportunity to get to know each other better. The settee in the Lighthouse Lounge in the Slieve was getting cosier too!

I enjoyed the godliest of courtships with Adrian. I remember early in our courtship, Adrian asked me if I would like to pray together with him, to which I boldly answered, 'yes'. I wasn't going to let him think I couldn't do that, despite my nervousness. There is a verse in Ecclesiastes 4:9 that says, 'Two are better than one'. I grew so much in my walk with the Lord during that time and was learning so much from this student for the Presbyterian ministry.

The first time Adrian met my parents will always stand out. We had left the Castle in separate cars as Adrian was heading on up to Ahoghill and Milly and I were meeting for tea. I introduced Adrian to my parents, then gingerly I tried to coax him away as I was leaving for my dinner date. I reached my destination and checked back with Adrian and discovered he was still at Mays Corner. It must have been going well!

## Missing you!

I knew Adrian was the man for me when he went away to France on an Oak Hall Christian holiday in August of that summer. I really missed him! Something else that was important to me was being absolutely sure I was in God's will regarding Adrian. Being a Christian was not enough, it had to be the right relationship—God's choice for me. I also was taking into consideration the fact that Adrian was training to be a minister and that I needed to be absolutely sure that this high calling and godly privilege to be the 'help-meet' of a minister was mine. I knew that difficulties could possibly lie ahead in ministry life as a couple and I wanted the full assurance of God's Word so that I would always have his promises to lean on. Did God give me his approval? *Absolutely*.

We were sitting together one afternoon in Adrian's home in Ahoghill which he shared with his dad. We were reading together

I love the verse in Song of Solomon 3:4 where it says, 'I found the one my heart loves.' This verse is so often used on wedding stationery and cards but what a beautiful picture of the Lord Jesus himself, and me, his bride. And, just as I had been preparing for three months for my wedding day to Adrian, making sure everything was perfect, how much more important it is to be ready to meet Jesus the ultimate Bridegroom. Why? Because he has gone ahead to prepare a place for his bride, the church, and he promised that he will come back again to take us to be with him. Then we will be with the Lord forever. There will be no separation anymore, no more appointments at the cemetery, and no saying goodbye to loved ones, what a comfort, what a comfort that will be to those who know and love him.

And so my heart was full of love as the car got nearer our wedding venue. The Lord with me, my daddy beside me, and Adrian waiting alongside our family and friends. Milly was ready to play, and Rev Brian Smyth was set to conduct his first wedding ceremony! Adrian and Brian are best friends so we were both overjoyed that he was both willing and very excited to marry Adrian and me that afternoon.

We said our vows to each other: Adrian promising to love, honour and cherish me, and me promising to love, honour and obey in the Lord. And yet, as I reflect now on the relevance of those covenant words, sickness has played its part in the fullest of ways, the most unexpected and unwanted of ways too. Marriage, in all its loveliness, is not shielded from the cares and struggles in this life. Yet I entered that marriage bond that afternoon with Adrian, with full hopes for a long and happy life together. Our confidence as a couple was—and still is—grounded and rooted in the Lord Jesus Christ, our anchor.

We walked out through the wedding ceremony suite for the first time together as Mr and Mrs Adger. As photographs were taken, our wedding guests enjoyed a golf-putting competition in the warm sunshine. Meanwhile, Adrian and I got a ride in a golf buggy around the course with Lynn Stanfield, our amazing wedding photographer, as she looked for those perfect picture opportunities. It was all over so quickly—the reception meal, the speeches, and the wonderful table quiz my brother David organised for entertainment afterwards.

## The honeymooners

We spent the next morning enjoying breakfast on the veranda of the golf club before heading to Mays Corner to see my parents and then onto Ahoghill to see Adrian's family. Adrian had booked our honeymoon—a week in the beautiful Algarve, Portugal. We stayed in Villamoura, a beautiful marina resort. Everything was just perfect. It was also important to us that we honeymooned somewhere where we could attend a church on the Lord's Day. Nearby was the International Evangelical Church of the Algarve. Adrian already knew the pastor and his wife, who also come from Northern Ireland, so we received a very warm welcome at the church.

We got to know faces around the marina as the week went on and formed a friendship with Manjit, who we still keep in contact with. While going out with Adrian, I already knew that I had met someone who loved the souls of men and women with a burning passion—and our honeymoon was most definitely not a week's break from his desire to reach everyone he spoke to. We were on our 'honey mission'. So, when we were approached to accept an invitation to a restaurant by the many waiters on the marina, Adrian was prepared with some Scripture leaflets of his own! I was not escaping either and soon it became a real adventure as we took turns in giving literature out.

Is this not what a godly husband and my spiritual leader should be practising? Always encouraging me, gently pushing me out of my safe, comfort zone, to grow stronger in my faith and love for the Lord and others. Two are better than one, as we read in Ecclesiastes 4, and Adrian and I are definitely better together than we would be on our own. We often speak together that we are a team in ministry.

It may not be for everyone to give out Christian literature to complete strangers, especially on their honeymoon, but we should still look for opportunities to witness to others as they come our way, with God's help. The company that we keep as Christian couples, the places we go, the things we say, and our conversation, all are watched by those looking at our lives day by day. I love Colossians chapter 3, so rich in godly instruction. Verse 12 says this:

> *Since God chose you to be the holy people he loves, you must clothe yourselves with tender hearted mercy, kindness, humility, gentleness and patience.*

And in verse 14:

> *Above all, clothe yourselves with love, which binds us all together in perfect harmony.* (New Living Translation)

Now that is a recipe for successful godly living. Imagine, as you get yourself dressed, and depending on the occasion, there is so much thought put into our clothing—careful consideration. We want to look right, feel comfortable, and yet it is more important each morning that we also 'clothe' ourselves in humility, love, patience, kindness, gentleness and so on because others do see what we are 'wearing'. Why is this all so important? Because this is the message about Christ in all its richness, filling our lives. We are representatives of the Lord Jesus himself (verse 16-17).

For most people, getting married involves some kind of upheaval, usually moving house or a change in other routine circumstances. In my case, there were three big changes. Just shy of forty years old, I left my home and church family for the first time, and my work in the Castle where I had served almost nineteen years. Adjusting can be difficult and unsettling. Change is not always easy—but sometimes it is necessary for our spiritual growth and development. We get very comfortable in our cosy lives, and even more so as we grow older. The plan for the newlyweds was to move into Ashford Lodge, Newtownabbey. Adrian was starting his assistantship in Ballyclare Presbyterian Church which was a short drive away.

## Chapter 4

# Finding a new role

I had no plans to look for another job at this time. Instead, my focus was my new husband, making a lovely home for us and trying to settle into the community. I fitted very well into the Abbeycentre shopping complex! I particularly loved a visit to the Marks & Spencer coffee shop as it was on the upper level and, on a clear day, I could see my beloved Mourne Mountains.

Coming from a Baptist church, attending the local Presbyterian Church with a different style of Sunday service and message was also a change and even a challenge for me. But I knew this was the Lord's plan and his new direction for my life, so I wanted to be part of the life of the church family. I knew also that the Lord was asking me to support, encourage and pray for Adrian in his role in the church in Ballyclare, as well as being involved myself where I could.

## Supporting role

I began helping in the Girls Brigade, using my baking skills, I helped with the Friday coffee morning, and assisted Michelle Purdy, the church deaconess when she needed me. I was voted onto the Presbyterian women's committee, which would prove invaluable when we moved to a new role in Clough and Seaforde. What was I learning? What was God teaching me as he led me out of my comfort zone? He was saying, 'Karen, "I have new plans for you, plans to prosper you, not to harm you, plans to give you a hope and a future".' (Jeremiah 29:11) Plans with Adrian, plans where the Lord would open up a door for a church where Adrian and I would serve after his assistantship was finished.

So, dear reader, I want to encourage you, if 'change' is where you find yourself at this present time, then embrace it, looking to Jesus to guide, lead and direct you step by step. Yes, it is difficult at times. No-one likes change—but he knows what is best for his children. Being in the will of God is paramount as we live day by day.

> *Trust in the Lord with all your heart and lean not on your own understanding; in all your ways submit to him, and he will make your paths straight.* (Proverbs 3:5-6)

So there is a submitting of our will to his will. That's where we can struggle with the flesh—when we try to do things our way and not his way.

God did open up a door for Adrian and me, very clearly and, more importantly, through his Word to us. I had said earlier that it was of upmost importance to me that I knew that God wanted me to be married to Adrian. Now I was asking God something else. I was asking God that he would also 'call me' to the work and ministry. I knew that Adrian was the one being called to be the minister but I also wanted to know a peace and assurance that it was also right for me. I believe that I am the 'help-meet' to my husband, in accordance to Biblical teaching on marriage. I love the way the New Living Translation puts it, 'It is not good for the man to be alone. I will make a helper who is just right for him' (Genesis 2:18).

Young ladies looking for a husband—and, maybe like me, the not so young—seek a man who is 'just right' for you. There is a saying that refers to finding 'Mr Right' and it is certainly the truth. The Bible calls believers to marry someone who belongs to the Lord (1 Corinthians 7:39) and furthermore 'we are not to be "yoked together" with unbelievers' (2 Corinthians 6:14). So, willingly marrying an unbeliever is to the detriment of our walk with the Lord.

Clough and Seaforde churches, to be honest, were not on my radar. I had just spent almost nineteen years of my life working and serving the Lord, just a few miles away in Castlewellan. Surely the Lord would not be taking me back the way I came? Adrian was not very familiar with the area, even though he had just spent the previous year driving regularly through Clough and Seaforde villages, en route to the Castle! However, he applied to be interviewed and I encouraged him one hundred percent. Soon afterwards, he was invited to speak on a Sunday. I went along to both services with him—first in Seaforde and then onto Clough. We were warmly welcomed by both church families and I was comforted by the fact that I was so near home. The next evening the church would make their decision, so we had to wait.

## Decision made

But the Lord is amazing and he told me that morning we were going to Clough and Seaforde Presbyterian Churches. I was reading my *Daily Bread* devotion and the Scripture was found in Deuteronomy 11:

> *Observe therefore, all the commands I am giving you* ***today****, so you may have the strength to go in and take over the land that you are crossing the Jordan to possess, and so that you may live long in the land the Lord swore to your ancestors to give to them and their descendants, a land flowing with milk and honey. The land you are entering to take over is not like the land of Egypt from which you have come ... But, the land you are crossing the Jordan to take possession of is* ***a land of mountains*** *and valleys that drinks rain from heaven. It is a land the Lord your God cares for; the eyes of the Lord your God are continually on it from the beginning of the year to its end.* (Deuteronomy 11:8-12)

I couldn't believe what I was reading! I knew the Mourne Mountains were nearby. I knew there were valleys and plenty of rain. I also knew that was a contrast to Ballyclare, where we were serving, which was a built-up town. It was not like the place from which we had come. I remember shouting upstairs to Adrian to come down, now! He was probably used to hearing that, but normally for dinner! I read the verses to him, quietly confident that God had let me know his plans for us. I remember saying to Adrian that I didn't have to wait until that evening to hear the decision, because we were going, and I was so sure.

That was a morning I will never forget in our home in Ashford Lodge. There were tears as we knelt before God completely humbled and broken. We took ourselves on a favourite walk that evening at Hazelbank Park, by the coast where we prayed and sang as we waited on a phone call. Sure enough, Adrian received a phone call and accepted a call from Clough and Seaforde Presbyterian Churches. What did God just do? He was true to his Word, he had indeed plans for us, plans for our future. There were other circumstances too that confirmed and directed Adrian's call to Clough and Seaforde but this story I share was so important to me, as I also wanted to know God's will for our lives. We are a team and we work as a team as we serve our Saviour.

## On the move

So I was on the move again. I had just settled into our 'wee nest' in Newtownabbey when I had to leave and try settle somewhere else. It broke my heart as I began packing up, watching the 'For Sale' sign being hammered into our garden. The relationships I had formed with people would, for certain, change and I was now thinking of a new house—the church manse—and new faces to get to know all over again. This time, though, I was on my home patch. I knew the area, it was a short drive home to Mays Corner and Sarah was nearby too. Previously, I was getting to grips with the busy roads around Newtownabbey and a trip home was always facing the gauntlet of the Sandyknowes roundabout in Newtownabbey and the Westlink in Belfast, where there can be a significant build-up of traffic. Now I was back to slow moving tractors and the occasional sheep on my run home to Katesbridge, but I didn't mind at all.

The church family were straight into action. They helped us move, they saw my tears as I left Ashford Lodge and they were there to help us unpack that Saturday afternoon in the manse outside Clough. There was a pot of soup, sandwiches and homemade treats. My head was there, but my heart was slow to catch up—and it's the strangest of feelings. Knowing you are where God wants you to be, yet with my 'my wee home' in Newtownabbey much in my thoughts.

We had almost a week to get settled before Adrian's installation and ordination service on the 19 June 2015. I remember a few other ministers' wives telling me to give myself two years to settle into the manse and they were absolutely right. I also wanted to concentrate completely on our new church families in Clough and Seaforde and supporting Adrian in every way possible. I always wanted to be active in the ministry with Adrian, to be a 'hands on' minister's wife. At times, the thought of it absolutely petrified me as I contemplated what lay ahead. Ballyclare I believe was my 'training ground' especially with Christine (Rev Bell's wife) who took me 'under her wing' for almost two years. I said on a number of occasions that the men got their training at theological college and that the wives had to jump in feet first! I knew God had also called me to be part of the work and, by his grace, I entrusted to him how I could be a blessing to others in the church family.

## Early days

I remember, in those early days, both of us trying to learn everyone's names. We had lots of other practical things to redo again—register with a doctor, change our address on all our post, and so on, but it was a really exciting time for us both. Folk from church were so friendly and called into the manse just to say 'hello' and so we felt really welcomed and loved from the very beginning.

I was praying about how I could be involved, what was right for me and how best I could use my God-given gifts to serve in Clough and Seaforde. I had a strong passion from the start that I would love to start up a coffee morning. This was taken by Adrian to his new

Kirk Session and all were in agreement that I could proceed. I was overjoyed, spurred on that my vision for our church family in the community was shared by others. We decided that the Old School in Clough was ideal for our new venture. It was a central location, and a neutral venue.

The aim of our coffee morning is to provide a safe, warm, comfortable, relaxed and friendly environment for everyone. We also have an opportunity to give to others financially at every coffee morning. We do not charge, but voluntary donations are greatly appreciated. The small team who freely help, and who are wholehearted in their commitment decide where we give the money gifts. We support a cancer cause once a year in September, but our priority is giving to Christian missions. We especially love it when we get a visit on the coffee morning from mission representatives. This is time where they can relax, chat and mingle with others on a one-to-one basis, sharing about their work, getting to know our folk too while enjoying a cuppa and a scone—pear and almond being a favourite. I also try at the beginning of each coffee morning to pray with my team and bring them a verse of encouragement from God's Word.

## Encouragement

There are many verses that come to mind, one is found in Hebrews 6:10.

> *God is not unjust, he will not forget your work and the love you have shown him as you have helped his people and continue to help them.*

Everyone needs encouragement in what they are doing—whether it's pouring a cup of coffee, offering a welcome at the door, a smile, a simple 'hello, how are you this morning?' can make all the difference in someone's life. So as we see in Hebrews 6:10, the Lord sees all this. He sees everything we do to help others—and not only help, but 'continue to help'. Loving our church family and community is not a 'one off' act of kindness rather it is a godly lifestyle! James 2:26

clearly teaches us that:

> *As the body without the spirit is dead, so faith without deeds is dead.*

So we are not saved *by* our good works, as it is impossible to work our way to heaven. Rather, our good works are the *evidence* of the life that has been truly changed by God's undeserved grace and mercy—as Ephesians 2:8-10 reminds us. And we all have an important role to play in the body of Christ (1 Corinthians 12).

I cannot share of my work in Clough and Seaforde without mentioning the women's ministry. I am blessed with amazing ladies in our church family. I have developed relationships and friendships with them and God has blessed me with some close friends among them. It is a tremendous blessing to have ladies that stand by me in the work, as I do believe women have an invaluable role in the life of the local church. I am learning constantly from women in our church who are faithful in their love for the Lord and others.

## Chapter 5

# Finding a heartache

Life was good—as the saying goes—for both of us. We were immersed in the work of the church family. Yes, life had its trials and concerns—but nothing compared with what was about to shake my world to its core.

I still remember that Tuesday evening in February 2017. The events stay etched in my mind, because my life changed forever on that February day. Adrian was upstairs. He called to me, and I could sense the panic in his voice. I knew something was wrong—he was clearly in severe pain—but we stayed calm. We waited a little while for the doctor to phone back but we didn't receive that telephone call and I knew I had to get him to hospital immediately. It was an anxious forty-minute drive to Daisy Hill Hospital in Newry, County Armagh. My Ade, as I call him, was in agony. We arrived safely and a wonderful paramedic attended us.

### In pain

As anyone who has had a trip to A&E knows, the wait seems to last a lifetime as others are called ahead of you. We were seen fairly quickly and that alone brings a degree of relief. The consultant was caring. He administered morphine and, once Adrian's pain began subsiding, I began to settle myself. Sigh of relief, panic over. I thought, 'Let's get home to bed and trust the suspected stone in his kidney passes.'

Little did I know, it was far from over. I was about to be plunged into the deepest trial I had ever faced. We returned to the hospital the next day, Adrian was much better than the previous evening but the consultant wanted to do a scan, just to check everything out. He sat us down and, as he did so, I caught sight of the cannula he was preparing. I knew it must be an indication that there was something more concerning that they wanted to investigate. The consultant proceeded to ask Adrian how his health was in general, and various other health related questions. By this point, my tummy was beginning to churn ever so slightly and my mouth was getting dry.

Then the consultant came out with it and said, 'Adrian, you have a large tumour on your kidney.' I sat there. I'm sure I had the most blank look on my face. Utter disbelief. I couldn't believe what I was hearing. By this stage, my tummy was doing absolute somersaults! It was the strangest feeling—I was completely overwhelmed with a million emotions flooding through my mind all at once. The consultant did remark, however, on how well we took the news. There was an element of surprise as he observed our reaction.

## Crying out to God

I was screaming inside for God to come help us—and Adrian was able, by God's strength in that moment, to gently but passionately share of the hope that we both had in the One greater than us, the Lord Jesus. The next thing I remember, the consultant was saying, 'Go get something to eat'. He had just delivered information to completely devastate me. The last thing I wanted was lunch.

Before we could leave, we had to wait on the results of a full body scan, and we praised God that the tumour was contained within Adrian's kidney. There was going to be a wait for a few weeks as our case was red flagged and we would be under the care of the renal unit in Craigavon Area Hospital, County Armagh. At this stage, we didn't know if the tumour was benign or malignant.

The two weeks waiting to hear the consultant's diagnosis and plan were two of the hardest, longest weeks of my life. I remember those next few days—I was completely heartbroken, I was crying constantly and I just couldn't pull myself together. I decided on the Thursday evening to go along to Girls Brigade in church. We knew life and serving the Lord had to go on for us during those next few weeks. I was standing there and my dear friend Maggie said to me, 'Karen, you've been crying.' She was right and I was absolutely broken inside. Then I remembered—I remembered God's Word to me that morning. I had been reading that morning from my *Daily Bread* app the story of Mary, Martha and Lazarus. The sisters had sent word to Jesus that the one he loved was sick. When Jesus heard this, he said, 'This sickness will not end in death. No, it is for God's glory so that God's Son maybe glorified through it' (John 11:4). I knew that the Lord gave that word to my heart that morning. His word just to me. Now I know that the words of people, words of comfort and expressions of kindness are indeed heartfelt and meaningful, but there is nothing anyone says that can compare to the Word of the Lord. His Word brings deep peace, joy and calmness to the most broken of situations. It's a word we can lean on confidently and with full assurance.

## Operation

So, a fortnight later, we heard the consultant's diagnosis and plan for an operation to remove one whole kidney, though we still didn't know whether it was cancerous or not. Some weeks later, on 7 April 2017, I held on tightly to that promise in God's Word, even as Adrian was wheeled into the theatre in Craigavon Area Hospital. I walked alongside him as far as I was allowed and I then did what I would normally do—phone my mummy.

Adrian had a time of recovery and we received the good news that the kidney operation had been a success. The tumour in the kidney was malignant, but the lymph nodes around the kidney were all clear so no further treatment was necessary. We would still be required to go for six-monthly scans for the next five years as a precaution. I was so relieved, I knew we could cope with that. I felt I could breathe again. Our nightmare was finally over.

After a time of recuperation, everything was getting back to normal in life and the church. Things were going so well. I wasn't even concerned about the looming scan in October. We decided to plan a holiday, back to Villamoura, which would fit in perfectly just after Adrian's first routine scan. I was so happy as I recalled our honeymoon in Villamoura. We even enjoyed a fantastic day with Les and Christina Drew from our Clough church who were also staying on the Algarve in Portugal at another resort. However, there was a slight bump in the week when we heard from home that my dad was in hospital with a slight heart attack—but mum assured us everything was fine.

On coming home, we knew we had to go back to Craigavon Area Hospital for the scan results. We were not concerned in any way, confident that the consultant's previous 'all clear' result would still be the case. Adrian had recovered well and we were getting on with life and moving forward with the work in our church.

## Bad news

Nothing could have prepared me for the earth shattering blow we were about to be dealt. The consultant sat beside us and all I recall really was his repetitive, 'I'm so sorry. I'm so, so sorry.' I was stunned, unable to speak as he delivered what could only be described as a death sentence. At the same time, parallel to the feeling of complete shock, was the peace of the Lord Jesus Christ. Psalm 34:18, a go-to verse for so many of us:

> *The Lord is close to the brokenhearted and saves those who are crushed in spirit.*

I was completely crushed, my heart was physically hurting as I tried to digest the information I had just received. Adrian and I were one, and when one hurts, we both hurt. I felt like I had cancer too. We called in with mum and dad on the way home, and shared the news with them as we knew they were anxiously waiting to hear from us. Also waiting for news from Adrian were his brother Neil with his wife Kate over in England, and Adrian's best friend Brian and his wife Pamela. Our nearest and dearest were also shocked to the core of their being. Our immediate family were told soon after, and Sarah.

We had less than a week to decide how we could best tell the other 'love' of our lives, our church family. We knew we had to share our burden openly and prayerfully with them. This was a huge blow to us as a couple and there was no way we could proceed forward without the support of those closest to us. We love the churches of Clough and Seaforde, our life and ministry is saturated in this community. Adrian shared his devastating diagnosis with those who had gathered for the evening service that following Sunday. There was utter disbelief at what they, our beloved church family, were hearing.

## Receiving the news

It was a massive relief to me too as I could be more open with the women whom I was closest to. We were already being supported in amazing ways prayerfully, but this was on another level completely. I have a friend in church who began sending me a message every night before going to bed and then first thing in the morning. Her sweet words comforted my soul. I was being loved through that early process. I was also spending time in those early diagnosis days with my friend, Maggie, who had her own path of pain due to the bereavement of a loved one. Having walked that journey with her as she grieved, I naturally turned to her as she understood my pain fully. We walked, talked, prayed, cried plenty and drank coffee—and I never felt I was a burden or inconvenience to her. Other friends would pray with me, others just listened to me, but they were there, and still are. We were seeing our church family regularly, some even on a daily basis. I know that, for me, it was vital for my well-being as I was still coming to terms with everything.

The support of our family was incredible. Neil was able to visit from England and, in between, was regularly in touch with us. My parents have been my rock, and Adrian and my dad have the loveliest relationship. I often pondered our call to Clough and Seaforde, our nearness to my family—yet Adrian's father was up in Ahoghill, even further away from us. I now know why. Adrian's dear father has gone on ahead of us to his eternal reward in heaven and that's far better for him. He was spared watching and seeing what Adrian is going through. I also thought it would be good that we would be closer to my family, so that we could care for them as they got older—but little did I know that it was actually them who would be caring for us.

## God's plans

God had it all planned out, what we were going through was always going to happen to us in the plan, purpose and providence of God. We said our vows to one another in July 2013 and the promise to love each other through sickness was now our reality. Nothing takes the Lord by surprise, ever. And even though Adrian and I were completely floored, the Lord is steadfast, nothing shakes him, he is sovereign over all. So I can trust him fully as he navigates us both through this ongoing trial. God still has a plan and a purpose for my life and Adrian's. He won't ever abandon, forsake or leave us. And so I have learned to trust him more and more each day—and it is a day-at-a-time journey that we are travelling. I think about cancer every day of my life. Every single day, it feels to me like Adrian and I are fighting a battle against a disease that wants to rob his body of good health. I never talk about Adrian's cancer, it's always our cancer, our scans, results, assessments and so on. I assure him constantly that he will never walk this path alone.

I have also found that continuing to focus my efforts in the life of the church has been a tremendous oasis for my well-being, working alongside Maureen, our Girls Brigade captain, and others in the Girls Brigade, leading the women's work, and the coffee morning. I have discovered even more that pouring myself into and investing in others, and listening to problems, worries and concerns that other people are carrying, has enabled me to look beyond my own heartache. I love the verse in Proverbs 11:25 that whoever refreshes others will themselves be refreshed. It is a profound verse that I often use in prayer.

Cancer has affected our relationship, as anyone who is suffering knows, and it touches the whole family. I know things are not the same anymore, and I often crave just to be normal again. I don't feel I am myself anymore. I live—yes, thankfully—by being carried along by the supernatural strength that the Lord is sustaining me with. But it is still an unwanted, uninvited trial on my part. No-one wants sickness at their door and that's a natural feeling. To get up in the morning, to go through the day and not to be living under the heavy cloud of illness is my heart's desire. We don't plan ahead anymore, I haven't flown on an aeroplane or travelled abroad in over two years, and even though I am content, it is more the feeling that cancer has robbed me of things and of places we would love to visit. We know aeroplanes are one of the worst places to pick up infection, and we should seek to be wise in our decisions.

## A solitary walk

I remember the summer of July 2019 and we were on holiday in the North Coast. It was early morning as I slipped quietly out of the bedroom, careful not to disturb Ade. I was glad I had packed my raincoat as the light drizzle met me on opening the front door of our rented apartment. I stepped out ready for my brisk walk. We were situated a five-minute walk from the beautiful promenade walk on West Strand beach, Portrush. I began taking in all the sights and smells around me. Joggers acknowledged me as they passed, and dog walkers greeted me good morning. But I was on my holidays, why was I walking by myself? It didn't seem fair to me that Adrian was too fatigued to get up and enjoy this beautiful walk with me. I was talking to myself which is not that unusual, and my mind was confronted with five words that stung hard: 'Cancer doesn't take a holiday'. It really hurt.

Cancer does indeed sting, and I can personally say it grieves me deeply. In 1 Peter 1:6 we do read about suffering grief in all kinds of trials and I can testify to this being absolutely true. Thankfully, we have verse 7:

> *These have come so that the proven genuineness of your faith—of greater worth than gold, which perishes even though refined by fire—may result in praise, glory and honour when Jesus Christ is revealed.*

Those five words were still churning over in my mind though and I knew I had to divert my attention, so I rang my mum. She talked to me until I reached my first destination, a coffee shop where I ordered my decaf, skinny, extra hot cappuccino. I proceeded back to the promenade, carry-out cup in hand, having had my mum for company on the other end of the phone. I do enjoy walking—it is a time when I spend alone in prayer with the Lord, and it is also a great way to just 'clear the head'. But, at times, it can also have the opposite effect, as it's during those times that my mind wanders. So I do love walking with others, normally around the lake at Castlewellan forest park or at Keel Point, Dundrum. I even have my 'adopted dog' Jack who I walk with, along with his real owner!

## Chapter 6

# Finding help during Covid-19

Christmas—that time of the year when coffee shops are serving their seasonal hot chocolate, toffee nut and gingerbread latte drinks. Homeware stores are filled with the sweet smell of cinnamon and winter spiced candles. The aroma of turkey roasting in the kitchen oven makes my mouth water. This is what Christmas smells like. No wonder it is my favourite holiday season. As I sat that November day in 2017, in the oncologist's office, trying to grapple with all the information she was feeding Adrian and me, she suggested we began chemotherapy treatment either before Christmas, or soon into the New Year. The consultant helped us make our decision by adding that before or after the holidays would not make much difference regarding Adrian's scan result. We had never experienced anything like this before and we listened as the possible side effects were read to us. I was squeezing Adrian's hand tightly as I tried to digest what I was being told.

We decided on the New Year to begin treatment, the sparkle of Christmas in my mind being tarnished and the possibility of sickness threatening us over the holiday period. I love to be organised, and do consider myself to be a bit of a planner. I love notes, exact details and I absolutely love lists. So where was Christmas going to be that year? I had never hosted Christmas before as we normally went to either Lynne and Denver's or David and Esther's house, all the family in tow, plus the two dogs, Nancy and Daisy. I wanted to have Christmas that year at the manse, as we really believed it was possibly going to be our last as a couple and we wanted to make it a special time to remember. The oncologist told us that the new drug Adrian was starting on only worked really effectively for a third of patients, giving us absolutely no guarantee of success. So I had to go for it with my Christmas preparations! The Christmas songs were on in my kitchen, Christmas movies played all day in the snug, and I was searching for the perfect gifts for my loved ones from us both. To quote the words of a well-known song, I was getting ready for my 'Last Christmas' with Adrian.

## Last Christmas?

Christmas came and treatment began, and we were doing well. About September time, maybe even earlier in the summer, I dared to dream that we might actually be blessed by another Christmas together. What would another year hold for us? I know our times are in God's hands (Psalm 31:15) and so I began to think about the miracle of sustaining grace that the Lord was doing in our lives as Adrian fought on with cancer. That was Christmas 2018 and another New Year was dawning. Would I get the answer to my heart's cry that Adrian would be healed from cancer? We did get another scan result that January, but I was dismayed and heartbroken as there was now a lesion in Adrian's liver. That year passed by too, and I can only cry out to God in thankfulness for the mercy he has shown us both by preserving our lives. And so another Christmas was glittering before me, with all the special events in church planned for that wonderful time of year when we celebrate the lowly birth of our Lord and Saviour Jesus Christ.

And so to 2020. How was my vision looking? How was I seeing things as the New Year lay ahead? January, the time of year when we make major life changes, when we plan to get fitter, thinner and healthier. My prayer for 2020 was the same as for the years previous: that this would be a new fresh start, with God working a mighty miracle and healing Adrian from cancer. Reports were starting to circulate in the news of a virus in China. Initially, I showed little concern for ourselves: we would certainly never be visiting China and I couldn't see how it could affect Adrian and me in Northern Ireland. We were settling into the work in Clough and Seaforde after the Christmas break, looking forward to what the Lord would have in store for our church families. Despite the relentless impact of cancer on our lives personally, both Adrian and I have a strong desire to continue serving our churches and community as best we can.

## Enter Coronavirus

Coronavirus was increasingly the only topic on the news and in social media. Early in March, Adrian and I were with a specialist cancer nurse, and he shared with us the strong likelihood that Adrian's next scan would be cancelled due to the expected influx of patients with suspected Covid-19 symptoms. I questioned his statement as it seemed impossible. He said it was coming and couldn't be prevented. He shared other things regarding this new virus and the possible implications for cancer patients like my beloved Adrian. Covid-19 was definitely now demanding my attention and I didn't like it one bit.

By the following week, things in our country had moved at a really fast pace. The new term 'self-isolating' was now being used and talk of having to spend weeks, perhaps months, separated from family, friends and loved ones. Our oncologist strongly advised us that we would initially have to stay isolating in our home for the next twelve weeks. This for our own good, and well-being, to protect ourselves from contracting the Covid-19 disease. I knew that if I personally became infected, I would most certainly pass the disease onto Adrian, who would have very little immunity to fight such a ferocious enemy.

I went to my local shop that evening, knowing that it would be the last time I would be there for at least the next three months. The enormity of the situation overwhelmed me as I pushed my trolley that I had disinfected the handle of around the aisles. Blinded by tears, I carefully went down my earlier planned written list, making sure I had missed nothing. There was a sense of peace that came over me that evening as I came home and locked the door behind me. The following week our government announced the beginning of a three-week lockdown on our nation. It was actually a comfort to know that the whole country was now doing the same thing. Naturally, everything had changed in our church life, no-one in living memory having any experience of such an event. Like most churches, we in Clough and Seaforde have been using the internet to continue the teaching ministry to our two fellowships and also those who follow us on Facebook.

## Isolation

I was missing my family and close friends from the start. I love company, and I knew I would most certainly struggle in this area. There have been quite a few self-isolating birthdays and mum and dad's wedding anniversary celebrations in our family—something that will resonate with most of us. The consultant told us that we were at an advantage by living in the countryside, and so I was thankful in a new refreshed way for the 'manse' home we live in. I began walking in our garden, so appreciative for what I had. Anyone who knows the beautiful Mourne area will know that we are so blessed to live in such a beautiful part of Northern Ireland. Sea, mountains, hills, rivers, lakes and forest, all on our doorstep, so to speak. Many of the small simple pleasures in life that don't even cost us anything had now been deemed 'non-essential'. I have not enjoyed the soft breeze or the smell of the sea for almost three months now and yet God has given me contentment and he does indeed give grace where it is much needed. As 2 Corinthians 12:9 says, 'My grace is sufficient for you'.

Adrian and I love hospitality and, on occasions, when we have had folk at our house for dinner, they remark that we have quite a big garden. I jest in response by saying that it's not my garden, but my field. Now this may be light banter on my part, but early in the lockdown, God challenged me regarding this. You see, what I had taken for granted previously, had now become absolutely everything to me. Before, it was all too easy to travel by car to my choice of walk, completely unrestricted in any way. Now I had 'my field' as my sole resource for walking, for somewhere to 'get out of the house', and to take my cup of coffee.

As Christians, we should be teachable, willing to learn, to grow, and to be corrected. Sometimes we also need to be challenged by God, and it is perhaps more difficult to bow our knee to his authority. I would never previously have entertained walking for an hour around the grounds of the manse, but now I was in a new situation. My undervalued 'field' during this lockdown has most sweetly of all become my new place to spend time with God in prayer. An hour passes easily as I walk in conversation with my Heavenly Father. God has taught me many things during this time: what is really essential and what is non-essential in my life. It's as if God has pressed the pause button on all our lives as we have time to re-evaluate our priorities. My 'field' is now my 'oasis' during this lockdown period.

## The next scan

To our surprise, Adrian was told that he would be getting his scan after all. We had little time to prepare emotionally for this, having just a week's notice. We were unsettled at the prospect of having to attend the Cancer Centre at Belfast City Hospital as this was beside the new Covid-19 Nightingale Hospital. We had masks, gloves and hand sanitiser, taking every precaution available. I was not allowed to attend this appointment, as I normally did, but instead had to wait in the car. The virus felt ever more real, tears fell as I sat opposite the hospital tower block, imagining the scenes in the ICU department and praying for those fighting for breath.

The result of that scan came by telephone the following Tuesday afternoon. I listened as Adrian relayed the consultant's conversation with me. A 'new small growth in my lung' pierced my whole being. For anyone who is living, or who has lived, this same journey of cancer, there is a flood of emotions like a fast flowing river engulfing every part of you. It is overwhelming, relentless and heart-breaking. But those are the kind of hearts God draws close to—the broken in spirit. A disappointing scan result is always hard to stomach, and it does take time to digest and come to terms with. The exceptional days we are living in make such circumstances harder, as we cannot be with our loved ones to comfort and hug us. That is when we snuggle more into the 'everlasting arms':

> *The eternal God is your refuge, and underneath are the everlasting arms.* (Deuteronomy 33:27)

Adrian and I have almost completed ten weeks of self-isolating. As our province and nation begin to emerge, baby-step regulations are being set in place. This glimmer of hope for people and families is greatly anticipated—but the sting in the tail is that it excludes at this time the most vulnerable and sick like Adrian. I crave the company of my family and friends, the smell of coffee shop cappuccinos, long beach walks, but this is the will and plan of God for my life at this time. I think of the song by local singer, Robin Mark, 'Jesus, All for Jesus':

> *All of my ambitions, hopes and plans*
> *I surrender these into Your hands.*
> *For it's only in Your will that I am free,*
> *Jesus, all for Jesus,*
> *All I am and have and ever hope to be.* [2]

## The future

How does the future look, almost halfway through 2020? Adrian and I have always taken one day at a time, not planning ahead as we cannot look too far. There is a saying on the lips of many in these days, 'This too shall pass', as there is a hopefulness that better and brighter days lie ahead. As Christians, we know that God has a good and perfect plan—as we read in Psalm 18:30, 'As for God, his way is perfect; The Lord's word is flawless; he shields all who take refuge in him.' We can trust God with all of our hearts as we continue through this bleak chapter in our world's history. Everyone, young and older, will have their memories and experiences of Covid-19 to take to their own grave. Those right on the frontline caring will remember how they bravely willed the sick on ventilators to breathe. Others protected the elderly residents in their care homes. The gifted at sewing made the much needed scrubs and face masks. Shop workers, lorry drivers and those in the food industry kept providing for us. Volunteers of many kinds, all helping each other.

Our cancer journey continues—but now with the threat of Covid-19, an invisible enemy with no vaccine. In a few months' time, the summer will have passed again, and another Christmas will be on my mind. I look forward to the gift of another Christmas in God's will and favour, to waking up on December 25th to say, 'Happy Christmas, sweetheart.'

What about Adrian? His turn to tell us more of his story.

Chapter 7

# Finding difficulties

People have said to me, 'your health is your wealth'. Healthy eating and living should therefore be our top priority. Exercise like jogging is essential to maintain and keep this wealth. People depend on their health for their entire well-being. However, what happens when your health is broken and you have been given no hope of recovery? Do you have any wealth whatsoever? Where is your true wealth? With my health severely affected by cancer, am I the only one in this kind of trouble in the country? Is my cancer diagnosis an isolated occurrence? Definitely not.

## Almost half

I was talking to a cancer nurse who shared with me that when she began this role in Northern Ireland, one in five of the population were diagnosed with cancer. Then it became one in four, then it became one in three. Now it is approaching one in two of the population. In Northern Ireland, 25 people per day are diagnosed with cancer, with 109 people per day being diagnosed in the Republic of Ireland.[3] Statistics reveal that 38.4 percent of people in United Kingdom will suffer from cancer at some stage in their lives. There are many individuals, families and friends devastated with the heartbreaking news. There are many who are struggling and in dark places as we have been. There are many in pain and in grief that I know nothing about. Many need to find hope.

If there are more and more people suffering with cancer, why is this happening in our country? Are we missing something? Why was I diagnosed with cancer? Is there anyone or anything to blame? Am I to blame? Is it my own fault in some way? Sadly, sometimes well-meaning people can offer unhelpful advice or even cures.

Some people say it is due to a poor diet. Since I have been married to Karen, my diet has been the best it has ever been in my life. Karen is a trained chef who uses fresh produce and cooks nutritious food. People say that cancer may be due to stress. Yes, there is stress in my life as a minister—but I have never been off work with stress in my entire life. I am thankful to God for the health he has given me and he has sustained me. Perhaps the cancer was due to a lack of exercise. Well I do spend considerable time in my study and I definitely could have exercised more but Karen and I enjoy walking in this beautiful part of County Down. We have walked up to Dundrum Castle, in Murlough National Nature Reserve, Dundrum, Castlewellan Forest Park, and Tullymore Forest Park and along the promenade at Newcastle to the harbour, and elsewhere. Could it be my genes? My mother took a clot and died at the age of seventy-two after suffering with Alzheimer's for seven years. My father took asbestosis and died at the age of eighty-nine, but this was due to working with asbestos earlier in life when the construction industry was not aware of the dangers involved. I don't believe the cancer was genetically passed on. There was nothing in my background or anything that I was doing, to my knowledge, that should result in such a cancer diagnosis. We don't know why I got cancer. Even the experts don't have all the answers.

How then did the cancer treatment work out? I began chemotherapy in January 2018 in tablet form using a drug called Sutent. Only one third of those on this treatment plan received news of their lesions shrinking. By the grace of God, I received good scan results in April and July 2018. In August, I was on holiday and I slept until after noon one day. I had my lunch and I still felt so tired that I climbed back into bed again in the afternoon. When I woke up, I was tired and weary of it all. I said to Karen that I felt that everything was getting too much for me and I was wondering whether I should resign from ministry in the church? Karen replied, 'No, I think you should keep going.' I was encouraged by her words. Then I read from Titus 1:2-3, 'the hope of eternal life ... which now at his appointed season he has brought to light through the preaching entrusted to me by the command of God our Saviour'. God spoke to me through his Word that he still had a work for me to do. I felt spurred on so I carried on in ministry and I am so glad that I did so.

In October 2018, I also had a good scan result. However, in January 2019, we received scan results that revealed that the tumours were now growing again in my abdomen. The cancer had also spread from my abdomen to my liver. The chemotherapy had stopped working. We had not expected that news and it really shook us. As we had in November 2017, we wept together and prayed. Once again, we shared our bad news with family, friends and our church family.

## New treatments

The consultant informed us that I would be going on a new treatment called immunotherapy. Immunotherapy seeks to stimulate our own immune system to attack cancer cells. It is increasingly becoming a frontline treatment in the fight against cancer. Professor James P. Allison and Professor Tasuku Honjo who pioneered this new approach to cancer treatment were awarded the 2018 Nobel Prize in Physiology or Medicine. The immunotherapy treatment kept the cancer at bay from January 2019 until the autumn of that year. I am thankful to God that I found the side effects of this treatment to be less severe compared to those associated with chemotherapy, and I had more energy on this new treatment. However, in October 2019 we were informed that there was a tumour continuing to grow on the abdomen despite this treatment, so I came off the immunotherapy. I then went onto a new chemotherapy treatment called Cabozantinib.

We have been dealing with so much uncertainty regarding my

health and treatment plan. As a result of these treatments I have received, my liver has now been adversely affected. The consultant thought it could be a side effect of the immunotherapy treatment or possibly of the Cabozantinib. Since my liver was affected, I had to come off the chemotherapy treatment. Then it was decided that I needed to be on a course of steroids to help the liver to recover. I began on a high dosage and, over a period of time, the dosage was reduced. The steroids gradually began to work. I was about to face another scan at the end of January 2020. However, as I had only been on the chemotherapy treatment for four weeks out of the last three and half months, I was expecting the worst news from the scan result. I was informed that I had not been on the chemotherapy treatment long enough to know if it was working. There was tremendous uncertainty regarding the future. There were fears and worries. What comforted us?

## Every day is given

Just before my scan result, on Sunday 26 January, we were singing a hymn at our joint evening service between Clough and Seaforde Presbyterian churches in Clough. The hymn, written by Keith Getty and Stuart Townend, was called 'My heart is filled with thankfulness to Him who bore my pain'.[4] I noticed a line in the third verse of the hymn:

*For every day I have on earth*
*Is given by the King*

The Lord spoke to me through that line. The next day, on the Monday afternoon, I reflected on this as I walked along the promenade in Newcastle with my wife. I thought about the fact that, in the midst of huge uncertainty humanly speaking, there is an even greater certainty that comforts me. Every day I live in this world has been given to me by my God the king. Who is in control? Who is in charge? Certainly not me and not the consultants or doctors.

Psalm 31:15 says 'My times are in your hands'. My times and

my entire life is in God's safe hands. God who reigns and rules all things from his kingly throne. I don't need to worry or be afraid. Instead, I can rest in these wonderful truths. Yes, we do not always understand God's ways; they are sometimes a mystery to us. At the same time, it is a great comfort to rest in the assurance that the Lord knows best. All that God requires of us is to do his will and follow *his* plan for our lives, not our own. The last two lines of the hymn are so appropriate and fitting:

> *So I will give my life, my all,*
> *To love and follow Him.*

Our hearts were filled with great thankfulness and joy as we reflected on these eternal truths that God revealed to us.

We received the results of the scan on Monday 10 February 2020. The lady at the Bridgewater Suite in the Oncology Department at Belfast City Hospital said to us, 'Good news.' The cancer had stabilised in my abdomen and liver. We were amazed and astounded. We were relieved and rejoicing. God had once again answered prayer in an amazing way, despite only being on the cancer treatment for four weeks out of the fifteen-week period covered by the scan.

## Praying friends

There is a particular day during that fifteen-week period—Tuesday 26 November 2019—that we remember well. The team of elders led by David Croskery and William McCall, the two clerks of session, called the two churches in Seaforde and Clough to fast and pray. That evening in Seaforde church hall, the church leaders and members came together to support us. The churches have been such an encouragement to us in their love and prayers for us. Hymns were sung in praise to the Lord. The people then came together to place their hands on us and pray for us and we sensed the presence and power of God among us. Graham Anderson, my father-in-law, brought a message from the Scriptures based on Ephesians 3:20, 'Now to him who is able to do immeasurably more than all we ask or imagine according to the power that is at work within us.' Graham was not aware that Karen and I read that verse from the Bible on the very day that we were given the news of incurable and inoperable cancer, back in November 2017. Almighty God is able to help us in our times of great need. God is always able to answer our prayers. We should never forget that nothing is too difficult for our God.

## Does God answer prayer?

At the same time, I want to draw your attention to a common and cruel misconception. Some people feel that if we simply pray hard enough and have enough faith, God will answer our prayers the way we desire—the scan result will be good and healing will come. And, if God hasn't answered our prayers and brought healing, it is because we didn't have enough faith or didn't pray hard enough. The problem with this idea is that the onus is all on us. I do believe that God works through the prayers of his people but, at the end of the day, it is not about us at all. Instead, it is all about God, bringing God glory and doing his will. When God does not bring the good scan result or the healing we desire and we are even more sick, it does not mean we have failed God or let him down or are outside of his will. We do know that there is a mystery to the will and providence of God. God has plans and purposes for us in times of health and in times of sickness. I will explain this further later in the book. God is not absent or remote from his people in their time of suffering. God is very close and near to us in love and mercy. What a faithful God we serve—as Psalm 46 reminds us:

> *God is our refuge and strength,*
> *an ever-present help in trouble.*
> *Therefore we will not fear* (Psalm 46:1-2)

I was led to share these verses at a funeral service on 13 February 2020, a few days after my scan results. I explained that, on one occasion, I was travelling on the ferry between Stranraer in Scotland

and Larne, County Antrim, one December evening some years ago. There was a severe storm in the Irish Sea and the wind and waves were battering the ferry in the high seas. Some people were staggering around the ship and the captain warned the passengers not to venture onto deck. It seemed as if we would be hours at sea, but finally the ship docked at Larne harbour and I walked down the gangway onto dry land. I was so glad to set foot on land again that I felt like kissing the ground. It was a huge relief. The port of Larne was the place of safety, the place of shelter, the place of refuge in the storm. Whatever kind of storm we face in life—and some storms may be very fierce—we are able to find a refuge and an ever-present help, if we flee to the Lord Jesus for mercy.

# Photo Gallery

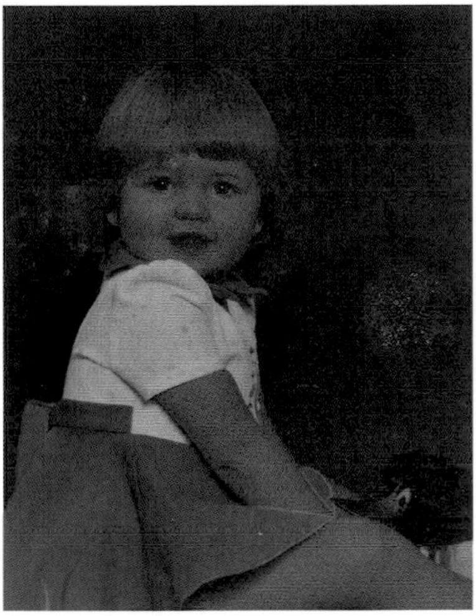

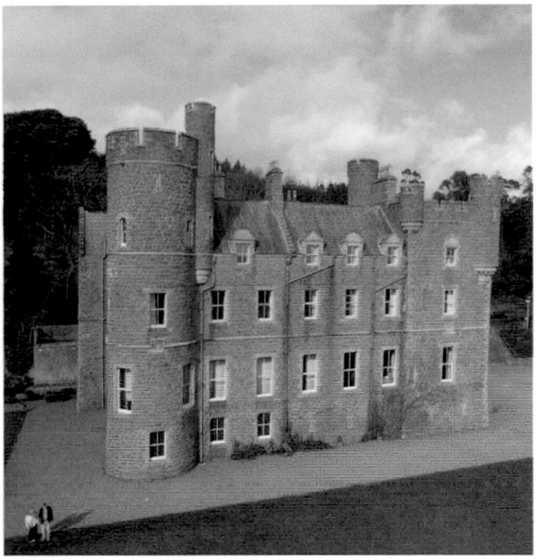

**Above Left:** Karen as a child

**Above Right:** Castlewellan Castle where Adrian and Karen first romanced.

**Below:** Karen's parents, Graham and Irene.

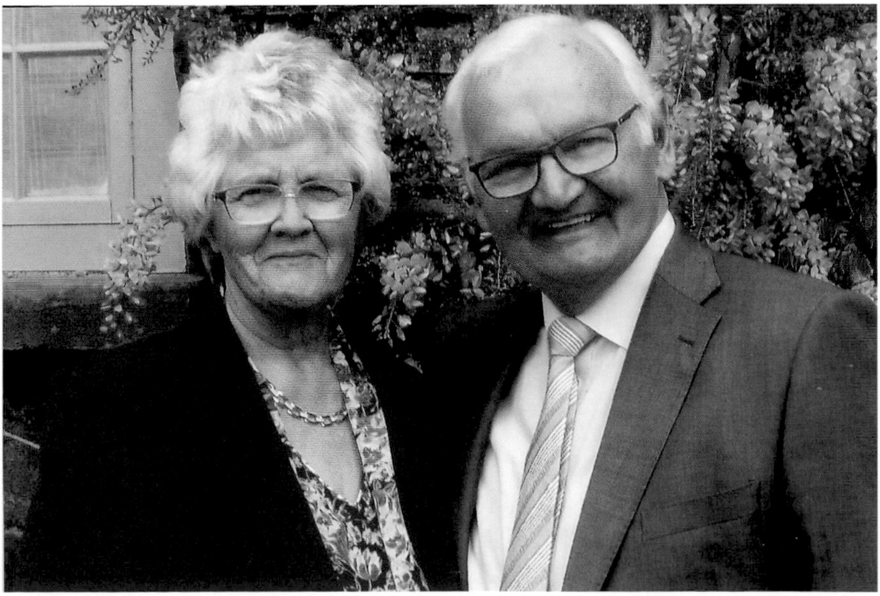

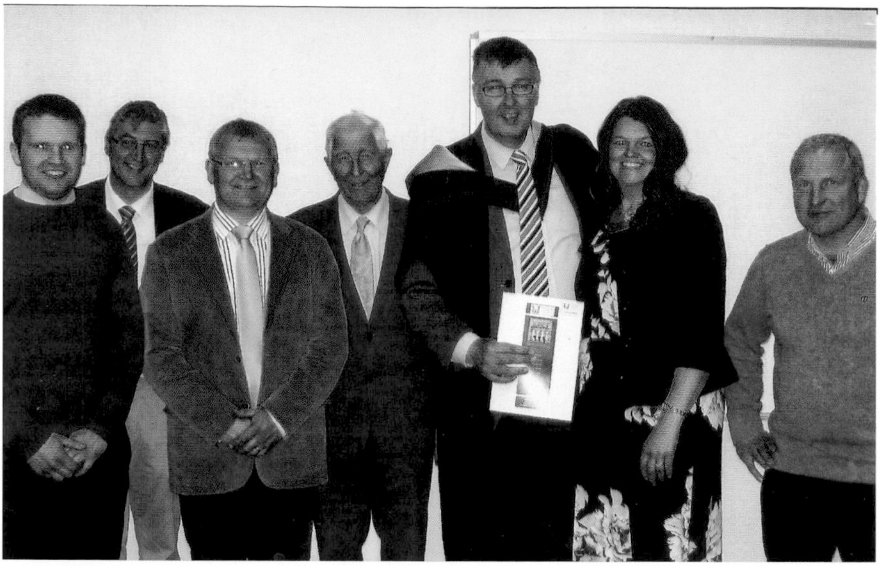

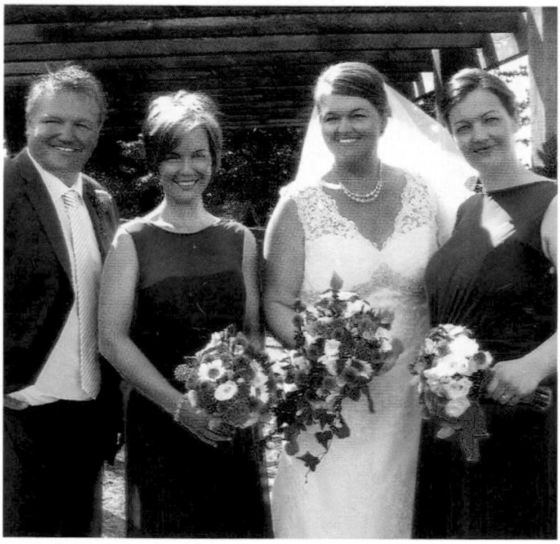

**Top:** Karen and Adrian (recently engaged) celebrating Adrian's graduation alongside Adrian's late father, William, and several friends

**Left:** Karen's siblings all scrubbed up for the big day: David, Lynne, the bride herself and Diane

**Below left:** The ring fits!

**Below right:** The honeymooners

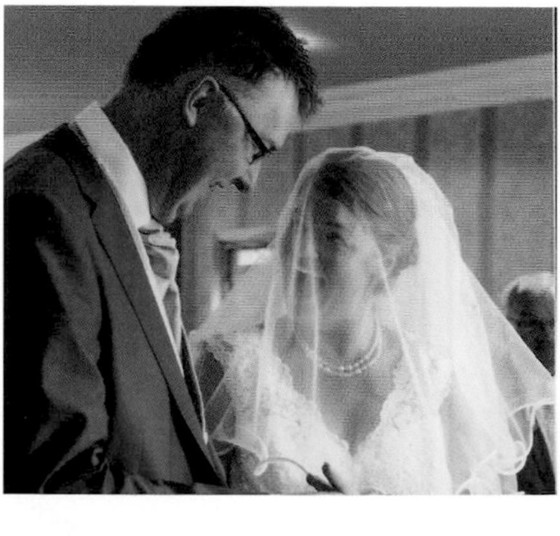

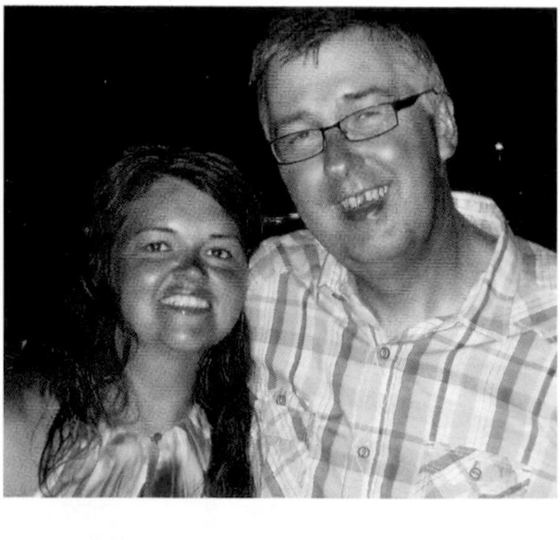

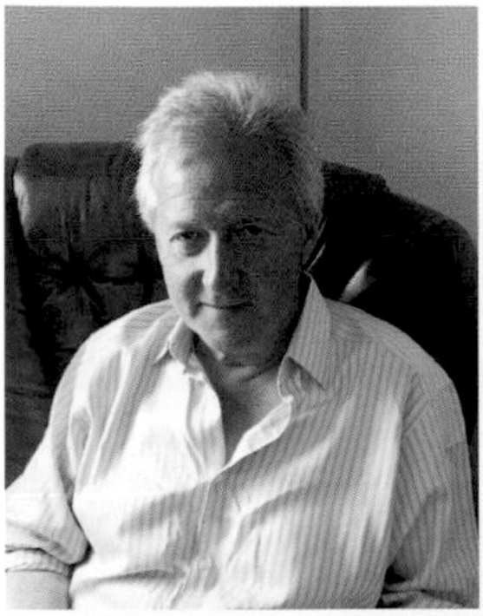
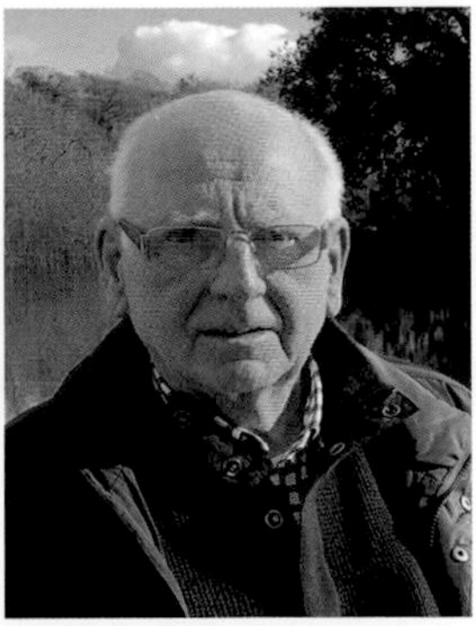

**Far left:** David Croskery, lead elder at Seaforde Presbyterian Church

**Left:** William McCall, lead elder at Clough Presbyterian Church

**Below left:** Karen with friend Sarah, on her wedding day

**Bottom:** Adrian interviewing Gary McDowell about what inspired him to write his songs, 'No Eye Has Seen' and 'Facing Cancer: Standing Together'

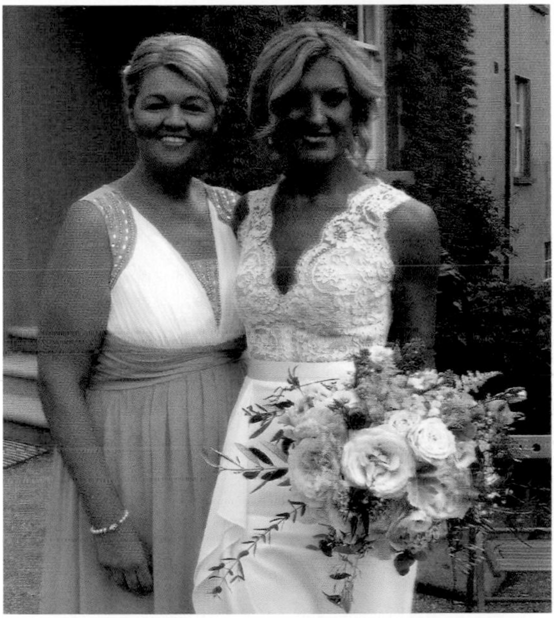

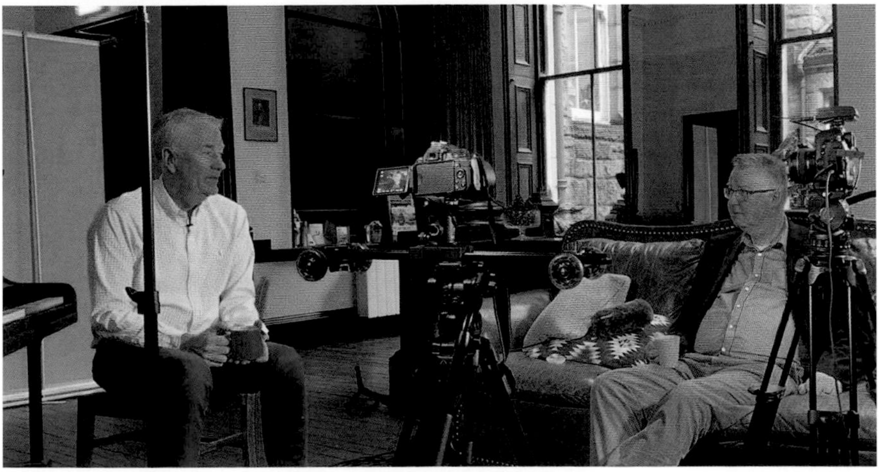

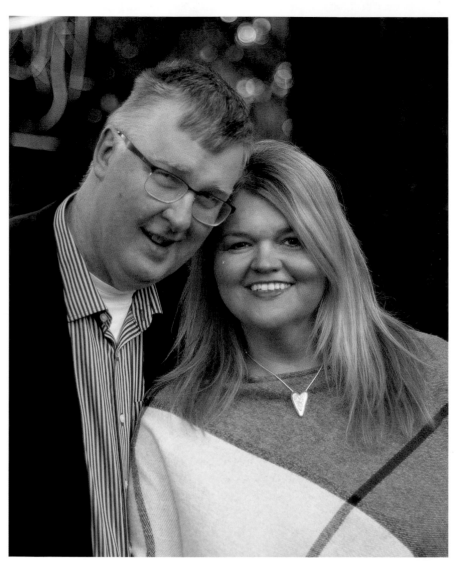

Adrian and Karen in February 2020

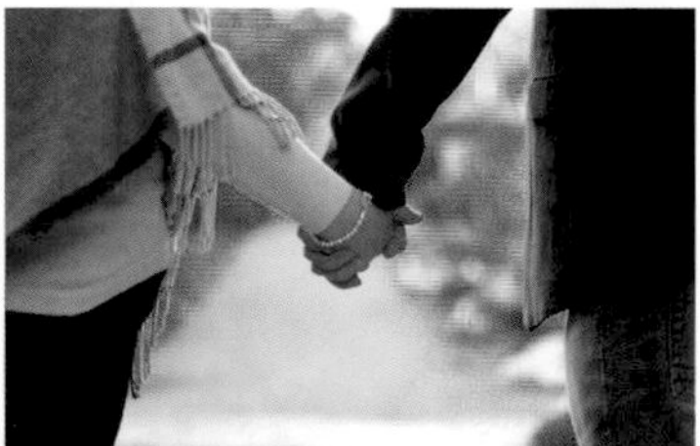

## Chapter 8

# Finding opportunities

Whenever people are given a bad diagnosis, it is such a devastating time and difficult choices have to be made. Some people go into denial—it does take time to come to terms with heart-breaking news. Some decide to keep the diagnosis to themselves for as long as possible and don't want others to find out. Perhaps they are trying to protect themselves or protect others from suffering. The danger here is that this may isolate themselves from others and cut themselves off from receiving valuable support that is greatly needed. Karen and I felt we would openly share this cancer journey with others. The Lord gave us the courage to be vulnerable and open about our struggles as well as our faith. We felt that it was good to do so. We also felt so weak and inadequate and we desperately needed the support of family, friends and our church family. We felt we could never carry this heavy burden on our own. So, we shared the burden with the Lord (Psalm 55:22, 'Cast your cares on the Lord and he will sustain you; he will never let the righteous be shaken.') But we also shared it with the Lord's people (Galatians 6:2, 'Carry each other's burdens, and in this way you will fulfil the law of Christ.')

### Testing

When incurable cancer strikes, our faith in God is really tested. We are confronted with our own mortality and that is very unsettling. Are we really ready to die or not? Are we unafraid or very afraid?

Where does our confidence lie in the face of death? These are challenging and important questions. If our faith in the Lord Jesus is genuine and real, it will shine in the midst of adversity. However, if it is not, then it is necessary to rethink our priorities and what we really believe. There is a heaven to gain and a hell to shun. Repentance and faith in the Lord Jesus Christ is absolutely necessary to be accepted by God and welcomed into heaven.

I thought my service for the Lord was over when I was given my first bleak diagnosis—but God had different plans. We have had wonderful opportunities to share with others the incredible comfort we have received from the Lord in our time of deep trouble. We have experienced the truth of 2 Corinthians 1:3-4.

> *Praise be to the God and Father of our Lord Jesus Christ, the Father of compassion and the God of all comfort, who comforts us in all our troubles, so that we can comfort those in any trouble with the comfort we ourselves have received from God.*

As a result of cancer, there have been many opportunities to share personal experiences as well as Scripture with others. We have cried and prayed with others—and they with us. We didn't realise it at the time, but having cancer has allowed us to better understand, empathise with and connect, in some small way, with the pain and experience of so many people and families. There have been many occasions for discipleship and counselling. There have also been opportunities to be involved in evangelism and mission as we were able to share with others the reason for the hope that we have. Rev Ian Harbinson brought this truth out so clearly in the seminar we attended at the New Horizon conference in 2019.[5] God's purpose is to use us as his witnesses even in the midst of trials.

## Temptations

One of the real temptations we face is to be so obsessed with our own needs, that we forget about others and ignore them.[6] This is a massive challenge as the needs of the cancer sufferer can feel all compassing at times. At times, we may be overwhelmed. Yet, when we reach out to others in love and with honesty, good and meaningful relationships are built and nurtured. As we pour ourselves into the lives of others, without realising it, we ourselves are helped and others are helped and blessed. We soon realise that every family has its own burdens and that we are not only ones who are broken and struggling. We are all in the same boat. We need one another. That is why we desperately need church, we need community. So, together we must seek the Lord's strength to persevere, to grow spiritually and be his witnesses before a watching world.

We consider it a great privilege to serve in the churches of Clough and Seaforde. It has given Karen and me joy and delight as, together, we have sought to love God and love one another. The Lord also opened a new door for me to share the gospel in a very surprising way. In November 2018, my cousin, Trevor Boyd from Ballymena, telephoned me to ask me how I was getting on? I explained that the Lord was sustaining me while I was on the chemotherapy treatment. I shared that I was fatigued in the mornings, yet on a Sunday morning I seemed to have more energy than any other day of the week. The Lord was giving me the added strength I needed to conduct worship in Clough and Seaforde Presbyterian churches on the Lord's Day. I explained that there were so many people praying for us, even people in different parts of the world. When we received the last scan result, the consultant mentioned that the radiologist had stated the word 'unusual' in her report. I said to Trevor that 'God does unusual things.' He replied, 'You should write a book!' I was taken aback and flabbergasted. I had never thought of writing a book in my life; it had never been on my radar.

## Write a book!

I didn't reply to Trevor's challenge and, in fact, ignored it altogether. However, that evening after I went to bed and fell asleep, something out of the ordinary happened. In the early hours of the morning, I woke up and a thought came to my mind: take a three-week sabbatical and write a book. I was shocked and surprised by that thought for a few reasons. First, I had never thought of taking any sabbatical leave before. Secondly, I had never any thought of writing a book before. Where did this thought come from? I wondered whether it was simply my own idea or was the Holy Spirit prompting me to do something new? I certainly couldn't simply ignore this. I didn't want to grieve the Holy Spirit or quench the Spirit—I wanted to walk and keep in step with him (Galatians 5:25). Then I noted that this felt like it a command: take a three-week sabbatical and write a book. If I ignored this, for me, it would have been an act of disobedience.

I needed to take action. The elders in Clough and Seaforde churches were informed and were supportive of the plan. Approval was granted by the church and I was off work on sabbatical leave from the 13 January until 3 February 2019. I had never undertaken such a project in my life but I really enjoyed writing a manuscript during those three weeks.

Dr Sid Garland, International Director-at-Large for Africa Christian Textbooks and also a good friend of mine for some years, agreed to be my mentor in the book project. He contacted two publishers to see if they were interested in publishing the book. However, both publishers turned me down. Given my precarious health situation (the cancer had now progressed to my liver) and the fact I had never written a book before in my life, it was understandable to be turned down—but disappointing. I thought to myself that this manuscript would never be published. Perhaps I had written it for my own benefit and that of my family. Finding a book publisher seemed a huge obstacle and an insurmountable problem. It appeared to be very unlikely that it would ever happen.

Later, Sid contacted me with some good news. He had 'bumped into' Tim Thornborough, whom he knew but had not met for twenty years, and Tim mentioned a freelance editor called Mary Davis. After I contacted her, she agreed to edit the material. What's more, Tim agreed to print it for us. Wow. We were now up and running.

The Lord had opened the door. The book would be self-published and the responsibility for ordering, distribution, administration and promotion lay with Karen and me. It did seem a very daunting task given my health and the fact that we had no experience in doing any of these tasks. At the same time, we knew a peace in our hearts and we knew God was in it all. As the line of the hymn by Kittie Louise Jennett Suffield says: 'Little is much when God is in it'![7]

Mary and Tim had worked together on other book projects in the past and it was such a joy and privilege for me to work with them on this one. Their dedication, advice and expertise were invaluable. The name of the book was chosen: *Facing Cancer: Standing Tall—One Christian's journey to finding joy*. As the book project neared completion, a date to launch the book in Clough Presbyterian Church hall was decided: Friday 24 May 2019. How many books should we order? Someone said to me self-publishing books don't sell. Someone else said to me there is a lot of selling in 500 books and I agreed with them.

## Attempt great things for God

After prayer, a quotation from William Carey, who is known as the 'father of modern missions', came to mind: 'Expect great things from God. Attempt great things for God.' I wanted to exercise faith and expect great things from God. I thought to myself: what would William Carey do? I thought 500 books was a lot to sell—but possible. I did not see 1,000 books ever selling, humanly speaking, as that was way beyond what I could envisage. By faith, we ordered 1,000 copies and Tim efficiently organised the delivery to the manse. I also thought there would be one book launch and that would be it. Then Rev Brian Smyth said that Trinity Presbyterian Church in Ahoghill, my home congregation, would be prepared to host a book launch. Then Alan Martin, who serves with the Belfast City Mission, also said that Belfast City Mission in the Fairview Road, where I use to serve, would hold a book launch. Being dear to my heart, I accepted Brian's and Alan's invitations. Would anyone attend these book launches? Again, I had no idea who would come along and how the launches would go.

To my great surprise, Clough church hall was packed, with 549 books being sold on the first evening. The Belfast City Mission and Trinity Church events were also encouraging and well supported and over 1,500 books were sold in the first three weeks. We were deeply humbled by the support we received. People also shared their own stories with me, sometimes with tears. My heart was moved and God continued to confirm that this was his doing all along and was not of me. More books from Tim had been quickly ordered and I was so glad that they arrived in time. Initially, I had thought that I would have only one launch but soon I was being asked to share my story and hold book launches in churches all over Northern Ireland. These unexpected opportunities showed that the Lord was leading the way. All I had to do was follow his plan. A door opened in County Monaghan, where my mum came from: Rev Stephen McNie was guided to hold a launch in a room in the Four Seasons Hotel. Rev Gordy McCracken was also led to hold a launch in Biddy Friels in County Donegal. I emailed Tim Thornborough and shared how things were going. He replied, 'Who would have thought that such bad news could be a door opening for the good news of the gospel. We have an amazing God!'

## Not the end, but a new season

After the bad news of incurable cancer, I thought I was finished, that this was the end, that death was imminent. It was a deeply troubling and unsettling time. We now realise it was not the end, but the beginning of a new season in our lives. In fact, there have been far more opportunities to share with others during my time of illness than in any other time of my life. More opportunities when I am seriously ill than when I had good health. How is that possible? How can that be explained? We know it is all of God's doing, it is all of God's grace—therefore, all the credit, all the praise and all the glory goes to God alone. We also should say that it is when we are at our absolute weakest, that God is often working the most. The Lord said:

> *My grace is sufficient for you, for my power is made perfect in weakness* (2 Corinthians 12:9)

And, earlier in 2 Corinthians:

> *But thanks be to God, who always leads us as captives in Christ's triumphal procession and uses us to spread the aroma of the knowledge of him everywhere.*
> (2 Corinthians 2:14)

I believe it is God who leads and uses ordinary, broken, bruised, suffering and weak people who love the Lord Jesus, to spread the lovely fragrance and aroma of Jesus Christ wherever we go. It is a reminder to us that God has purposes for our lives when we are healthy and when we are sick. We are so very thankful, grateful and full of gratitude to the Lord for we do have an amazing God.

## Questions and answers

In Ballynahinch Baptist church, after I had shared the message at the Sunday evening service, the pianist quoted the Heidelberg Catechism. I was intrigued and needed to find out more. I discovered that this confession was not written a few weeks ago or a few months ago or a few years ago—but in 1563. The Lord spoke to me through what was said in the catechism.

> ***Question 1:*** *What is your only comfort in life and death?*

What a profound question. What a very important question. What do I treasure in life and death so that I am fully prepared and unafraid to die? Is it my church attendance? Is it my prayers? Is it my Bible reading? Is it my giving to charity? Is it the fact that I am a good person and do not do anyone any harm? So many find comfort simply in their possessions, in their position, in their power, in their family and in themselves.

However, the answer the Catechism confession gives is this:

> ***Answer:*** *That I am not my own, but belong with body and soul, both in life and in death, to my faithful Saviour Jesus Christ. He has fully paid for all my sins with his precious blood, and has set me free from all the power of the devil. He also preserves me in such a way that without the will of my heavenly Father not a hair can fall from my head; indeed, all things must work together for my salvation. Therefore, by his Holy Spirit he also assures me of eternal life and makes me heartily willing and ready from now on to live for Him.*

Kevin DeYoung comments:

> *We can endure suffering and disappointment in life and face death and the life to come without fear of judgment, not because of what we've done or what we own or who we are, but because of what we do not possess, namely our own selves.*[8]

It is a question of identity. We do not belong to ourselves, but to Jesus Christ, when we are united to Christ by faith. Jesus died on the cross of Calvary and paid the price to set us free. 1 Corinthians 6:19-20 says, 'You are not your own; you were bought at a price.'

## The Shepherd and his sheep

Some of us will know and love that song by Norman Clayton, 'Now I Belong to Jesus':

> *Now I belong to Jesus*
> *Jesus belongs to me*
> *Not for the years of time alone*
> *But for eternity.*[9]

What a great comfort this is to the believer. Whatever circumstances we face, we have a Saviour and Shepherd in the Lord Jesus.

On one occasion, I called in to the home of a shepherd outside Ballymena, who owned some pedigree sheep. It was a lambing season and there was a fox prowling around the fields. The shepherd was aware of the danger this posed for his flock. There was a lamb that was born sickly and weak, so the shepherd went out into the field to rescue it. Then he brought it into the safety and warmth of his own home. There was a fire burning in kitchen and there was a basket by the hearth which the cat normally lay in. The cat was pushed out of the basket and the lamb was placed in the basket. The shepherd took a baby's bottle and filled it with milk. He then stooped down and fed the lamb. Over time, the lamb grew stronger and it became a pet lamb. The shepherd's children played with the lamb and it was treated as one of the family. We see the love the shepherd had for the lamb in his flock and how he protected it from the cruel fox. How much more does the Lord Jesus love us! Jesus said in John 10:11,

> *I am the good shepherd. The good shepherd lays down his life for the sheep.*

Jesus alone laid down his life for us on the cross of Calvary. As the Heidelberg Catechism states, he has 'set me free from all the power of the devil'. Jesus alone is able to protect us from the cruel fox, the enemy of our souls, the devil. Jesus alone is able to bring us to the safety of his home in heaven.

> *Surely your goodness and love will follow me all the days of my life, and I will dwell in the house of the Lord forever.* (Psalm 23:6)

## Singing for joy

During the service to mark the book launch in Clough, Denver and Lynne Wilson sang, as well as Keith and Karen Lindsay. The church praise group played their instruments. The Lord spoke to me at that service about the importance of praising the Lord not only when everything is going your way but also in the storms of life. The idea came about of producing a CD with singers praising the Lord in song, and with my story of God's amazing grace included.

Who would be the singers? I was definitely ruled out! It would have been 'Top of the Flops'! Who would possibly be interested? While I was attending Keswick Portstewart Conference in July 2019, I met Gordy McCracken. I knew Gordy well as we were colleagues with the Belfast City Mission some years earlier and we are now in ministry together in the church. He was excited by the singing project. Then I met Gary McDowell at the New Horizon conference at Coleraine in August 2019. I knew Gary as we met as students at Belfast Bible College in 1991 and we serve together in the church. Gary was also keen to be involved.

I felt that while living with cancer, I should be singing with joy and encouraging others to praise God for who he is and what he has done. We should never stop singing, whatever the circumstances of our lives—whether we are on the mountaintop or in the valley. Cancer is not good, but even in such storms we should still count our blessings and name them one by one and it will surprise us what the Lord has done.[10]

## Title track

I met Roy Rainey at the same New Horizon conference at Coleraine—he has expertise as a recording engineer and music producer. He was keen to produce the CD in his recording studio in Portstewart. It was all falling into place. Eight songs were recorded and other singers were involved. Gary wrote a new song that autumn called, 'Facing Cancer: Standing Tall' which became the title tract for the CD. The CD was launched in a bookshop called 'The Secret Place' in Ballyclare in mid-December 2019. The managers of various bookshops also came on board for this project and were so encouraging and helpful. We now have a greater appreciation for the ministry that goes on in Christian bookshops in towns and cities in Northern Ireland and beyond! They not only provide invaluable resources to the churches but, when churches are closed, during the day, when someone is in need, there is always a listening ear to be found in the staff in these shops.

Soon after, came the idea of producing a music video for Facebook and YouTube so that others could hear some of the songs on the CD and be encouraged in their faith. Jonny Sanlon, a good friend with expertise as a videographer, suggested using Castlewellan Castle as a venue which was a tremendous idea, given Karen's and my links with the place. Andrew Forson, the manager of the Conference centre, kindly granted us permission to use the building. Videos for two of the songs 'Facing Cancer: Standing Tall' and 'No Eye Has Seen' were produced and the story behind these songs were then recorded. They were released on our church Facebook page and YouTube channel in March 2020 and on the church website in May.[11]

## God's grace to Africa

We decided that the profits we make on the CD and the book will be given to Kisakye Ministries in Uganda. This ministry was set up by Christopher and Hannah Brown, who belong to our church family in Clough. *Kisakye* means God's grace. This is a Christian ministry in Uganda, empowering families by providing them with housing, education and farmland to encourage lasting self-sustainability. Christopher and Hannah have recently returned to Northern Ireland after a five-month mission trip to Uganda. During that time, they provided solar powered Bibles in the Luganda language for people and were doing discipleship work with men, women and teenagers. Christopher was also preaching regularly and sharing the gospel in local churches. It is a wonderful ministry—you can find out more in the Facebook page for Kisakye Ministries or on their Instagram account.[12]

The Lord continued to surprise us with unexpected avenues of service. At the beginning of July 2019, David Thompson telephoned to ask if I would be interested in sharing my story on 'The

Nolan Show' on BBC Radio Ulster. After the conversation, Karen and I discussed it, and she said, 'Go for it!' We prayed about it and I agreed to do a radio interview. A few days later, I was interviewed by Vinny Hurrell. Vinny was easy to talk to and sympathetic towards me because of the troubles I was facing. The Lord helped me in my time of need. I was also interviewed by journalists from the *Belfast Telegraph* as well as the *Newsletter* newspaper and had articles published in many local newspapers. I am reminded of 1 Peter 3:15, 'But in your hearts revere Christ as Lord. Always be prepared to give an answer to everyone who asks you to give the reason for the hope that you have. But do this with gentleness and respect.' I am so grateful for the privilege of simply sharing the reason for the hope that I have in the Lord. We are to be signposts, pointing people away from ourselves and to the Lord.

## Quality time with Karen

The year provided opportunities to spend special and quality time with my beautiful wife Karen. Karen is beautiful on the outside and inside—and I love her dearly. In all of the world, God could not have given me a better wife than Karen. She is a wife of godly character.

> *A wife of noble character who can find? She is worth far more than rubies. Her husband has full confidence in her and lacks nothing of value. She brings him good, not harm, all the days of her life.* (Proverbs 31:10-12)

I am so grateful to the Lord for Karen who enriches my life and brings me so much good. She has had an extraordinary amount to cope with and she has been so amazing. So practical on the one hand, and so full of faith and compassion on the other. I would be lost without her. We have been building new memories together as we have holidayed, exploring different parts of Northern Ireland, especially the North coast.

On one occasion, we travelled to Ballybay, County Monaghan,

and stayed with Francis (my cousin) and Eleanor Wilson. We had a fantastic time together and their hospitality was amazing. They run a bed and breakfast guest house in Ballybay. We were shown around the farmhouse just outside the town of Ballybay where my grandparents, Robert and Elizabeth Cuming, lived. We saw the primary school my mother Eileen attended, as well as the church. When my mother was around eleven years old, the family moved north and bought a farm in Lylehill, near Templepatrick. Then a few years later, my grandparents emigrated to Australia, as did their sons, Harold, Cecil and Rex. The other son, Tommy, left Ireland to live in Coventry in England, and so did their daughter, Alice. My mum, Eileen, was the only one of her family to remain in Ireland. She met my father, William Adger—they were married and moved to Ahoghill, outside Ballymena and, as they say, the rest is history. It was wonderful to share this with Karen and have a trip down memory lane together. It is good to look forward to holidays, having special breaks and go out for coffee together. Time with family is precious and invaluable.

## Facing a new year

In many ways, 2019 was a very tough year in our lives because living with cancer, having many hospital appointments and dealing with the side effects of immunotherapy, followed by chemotherapy, was not easy. At times, it was a real struggle to keep on going and, at times, we felt overwhelmed—especially when the news was not good from the hospital. At the same time, as I look back on the year, I see it as the best year of my life due to the many opportunities to share the gospel and be a witness for Jesus Christ.

On the way to a hospital appointment after Christmas 2019, Karen shared her idea to have a get-together of the church families in the two churches on New Year's Eve, to finish the year together. The team in Seaforde Presbyterian church were contacted and plans quickly fell into place. Many families came along to the church hall. We had some games together and a great time was had by all. Afterwards, we had a delicious supper followed by a short service which began at 11:38 pm. My plan was to finish the service just before 12 midnight and see in the New Year counting down the last seconds of the old year and listening to Big Ben chime in the New Year using technology. However, the service was slightly longer than expected, so instead, we sang the first verse and chorus of the song by William J. and Gloria Gaither, 'God Sent his Son, They Called Him Jesus' in the last few minutes of 2019. Then, in the first few minutes of 2020, we sang the third and final verse—'And then one day I'll cross the river'—followed by the chorus. The chorus is as follows:

> *Because He lives I can face tomorrow;*
> *Because He lives all fear is gone;*
> *Because I know He holds the future,*
> *And life is worth the living just because He lives.*[13]

Looking back, there is no better way of leaving an old year behind and beginning a new year than singing the praises of the Lord. Rejoicing that he is alive, that he holds the future safely in his hands and that, therefore, in light of that, life is really worth the living.

## Chapter 9

# Finding comfort

When the word 'providence' is mentioned, some people will think of a city in the United States of America. Providence is the capital city of the US state of Rhode Island. There is another occasion where the word is used—*The Westminster Confession of Faith*, chapter 5, section 1—which reads:

> *God the great Creator of all things doth uphold, direct, dispose, and govern all creatures, actions, and things, from the greatest even to the least, by his most wise and holy* ***providence*** *according to his infallible foreknowledge, and the free and immutable counsel of his own will, to the praise of the glory of his wisdom, power, justice, goodness, and mercy.*[14]

God not only is the Creator of all things including the earth, he also is the Sustainer of all things. Providence emphasises the fact that God governs and controls all things by his mighty power. He is sovereign and he has absolute authority over everything he has made. I was sharing my life story including my battle with cancer at a meeting in June last year in Mourne Presbyterian Church in Kilkeel. It was a joint service along with Kilkeel Presbyterian Church, as the minister Stephen Johnston also brought their midweek meeting along. Afterwards, the minister of Mourne, William Bingham, said to me, 'God's sovereignty is our sanity.' How true that is. It is because God is in control that I am encouraged and comforted.

I am living with much uncertainty as I wait for the continual round of three-monthly scans to find out if my cancer is shrinking or is remaining the same or is growing. I have no idea what the outcome will be. Facing a scan at the hospital is fine but facing the result of the scan is altogether different as it may bring anxiety, even fear and dread. Given the fact that my cancer started in my kidney, moved to my abdomen, then to my liver and now to my lung, where is it going to move to next? When I am going to be in such great pain that it will bring an end to my vocation as a minister? How long do I have to live? Is my cancer an accident or is it due to bad luck or is it due to 'bad karma' or is it the result of a chance spreading of malignant cells to organs in my body. If that is the case then there is no comfort for me, for there is no reason or purpose for my suffering. My suffering holds no meaning and it is futile for me to endure it. I may as well throw in the towel and give up the fight.

## Asking "Why?"

God's Word allows us—and in fact, it encourages us—to voice our longings and our questions: 'Why, Lord?', 'How long, O, Lord?' Sometimes we don't even know what to pray. As Romans 8:23 says, we 'groan inwardly as we wait eagerly for our adoption to sonship, the redemption of our bodies.'

However, when I understand that God, who is my Father in heaven, is providentially guiding me step by step in my life, when I understand that he is fully in control, then I am comforted and helped. I know God has a greater plan and higher purpose, even when I do not understand it all, and so I am able to trust fully in his wise and loving providence. Whatever the outcome of the scans—and I do long for a good outcomes—I know my future is safe and secure in God's hands. This does not take away the stress, the pain, the suffering or the grief but I am helped, strengthened in faith, encouraged and have real hope. I am able to know God's peace that surpasses all human understanding:

> *And the peace of God, which transcends all understanding, will guard your hearts and minds in Christ Jesus.*
> (Philippians 4:7)

I am also able to experience joy on the journey and in the battle: Nehemiah 8:10 says, 'the joy of the Lord is your strength'. Therefore, I will persevere and not give up my faith. God has purposes for us when we are healthy and when we are sick. In fact, I will cling even more tightly to the promises of God in Scripture and to my Saviour Jesus Christ in the midst of the trial. God is working his plans and his purposes in my life—not my measly little plans or purposes. No cancer is able to thwart the plans and purposes of God for my life in fact it is part of those plans.

Philip McKelvey, a colleague in ministry, wrote this, 'True faith rests upon God regardless of whether or not he grants our request for healing. It accepts his sovereign will, it rests on the providence of God.'[15] We rejoice that, unlike ours, God's plans will always work out, they will always come to pass. In Ephesians 1:11, Paul writes:

> *In him we were also chosen, having been predestined according to the plan of him who works out everything in conformity with the purpose of his will.*

Romans 8:28-30 reminds us what God's good purposes are for his people:

> *And we know that in all things God works for the good of those who love him, who have been called according to his purpose. For those God foreknew he also predestined to be conformed to the image of his Son, that he might be the firstborn among many brothers and sisters. And those he predestined, he also called; those he called, he also justified; those he justified, he also glorified.*

Not everything that happens us is good, far from it, yet we are confident that God works in all the circumstances of our lives to accomplish his good purpose. That 'good' purpose is twofold: a) that we might spiritually grow into the image of his Son, that we might become increasingly more like Jesus in his wonderful character; b) that God who *began* the work in us will *complete* that work in us by bringing us one day to final glory.

> *All the days ordained for me were written in your book*
> *before one of them came to be.* (Psalm 139:16)

I looked up a website to discover that I am 20,808 days old at present! I will not live one day longer or one day shorter than God has planned for me... I will not die one day, or one hour, or one minute, or one second *before* my time—nor will I die one day, or one hour, or one minute, or one second *after* my time. I will not die before God's appointed and planned time. My God the King has my life all planned out in advance. I acknowledge there is a mystery to the providence of God and I do not understand it all, but I accept it and believe it. I praise God for his loving providence.

## The choice we must make

I was deeply moved by a song that I sang at the Westminster Fellowship Conference in Ballymena. The verses ask a series of questions:

> *Who has held the oceans in His hands?*
> *Who has numbered every grain of sand?*
> *Kings and nations tremble at His voice,*
> *All creation rises to rejoice.*
>
> *Who has given counsel to the Lord?*
> *Who can question any of His words?*
> *Who can teach the One who knows all things?*
> *Who can fathom all His wondrous deeds?*
>
> *Who has felt the nails upon His hands*
> *Bearing all the guilt of sinful man?*
> *God eternal, humbled to the grave*
> *Jesus, Saviour, risen now to reign!*[16]

The refrain is again and again and again:

*Behold our God seated on His throne*
*Come, let us adore Him*
*Behold our King! Nothing can compare*
*Come, let us adore Him.*

This hymn draws from Isaiah 40:12-14. God is sovereign—but he is not the author of sin. He is never to blame for the evil that we see all around us in this world. Romans 5:12 says, 'Therefore, just as sin entered the world through one man, and death through sin, and in this way death came to all people, because all sinned'. People are still fully responsible for their actions and reactions. We are responsible for our sin and wrongdoing. We are accountable to God for how we spend our lives. We have choices to make—and the decisions that we make really matter. Charles Spurgeon said that the responsibility of man and the sovereignty of God are like two railway tracks that run very nearly parallel, side by side, and they never meet in this life—but they do meet in eternity.[17] There is an apparent paradox and tension between these two Biblical principles—yet both are true at the same time.

## Why prayer matters

Where does prayer fit into this? Does it matter if we pray or not? God has eternal purposes and these plans will come to pass in God's appointed time, but he uses 'means' or 'ways' to bring about these purposes. One of the ways God uses to bring about his plans in this world are the prayers of his people. The Lord Jesus himself was constantly in prayer. He taught the disciples about persistence in prayer and prayed often. For example, we read in Luke 6:12-13 that:

*Jesus went out to a mountainside to pray, and spent the night praying to God. When morning came, he called his disciples to him and chose twelve of them, whom he also designated apostles.*

So, before the important work of selecting the twelve apostles, the Lord Jesus spent the whole night in prayer. Jesus prayed on the Mount of Olives in the Garden of Gethsemane in the evening before His death on the cross of Calvary:

> *Father, if you are willing, take this cup from me; yet not my will, but yours be done.* (Luke 22:42)

The Lord Jesus is not only the Saviour of those who believe, he is also our example to follow. Prayer therefore is of paramount importance.

> *Is anyone among you in trouble? Let them pray … Is anyone among you sick? Let them call the elders of the church to pray over them.* (James 5:13-14)

Praying to God is the correct way, the right way, to handle suffering and difficulties. This should be the natural response for the believer. The hymn reminds us:

> *What a friend we have in Jesus,*
> *All our sins and griefs to bear!*
> *What a privilege to carry*
> *Everything to God in prayer!*[18]

Of course, we do need to pray as the Holy Spirit leads us. Let us praise the Lord in prayer for the personal relationship and friendship we enjoy with the Lord Jesus. That is an awesome privilege. Sometimes prayer means confessing our sins, sometimes it means asking God what he is teaching us through the trial. Certainly we do need to apply God's Word to our lives, as we humble ourselves and bow under its authority. Submitting to the truth does bring wellness and wholeness to us—a spiritual and inner healing that lifts us up.

> *Truth brings a 'healing' of its own … the search for inner healing is a valid one. As the gospel transforms lives, bringing a yet deeper repentance, so the healing of Christ*

*reaches deeper into our being, enabling us to forgive and find forgiveness.*[19]

Sometimes we need to ask God to help us to come to terms with the new situation and to accept his will. Our delight is in doing God's will. Powlison—who had cancer himself—also urges Christians with cancer to ask others to pray that, in the midst of our cancer, we would 'experience peace, patience, growing faith, and the inclination to love others.'[20]

## Boarding for heaven

I remember a minister shared a story with me: an aeroplane was due to depart from Belfast International Airport, bound for heaven. Places were available for anyone who wanted to take the flight. It was due to leave on Monday morning at 9 o'clock. He asked the question, 'How many people would choose to be on board? Would the plane be full or half full or empty?' He replied, 'Practically no-one would be on the plane—it would be empty.' He said, 'Everyone *wants* to go to heaven—but *not now*, not today.' How true that is. God has placed a desire within those who love him to live in the context of close relationships with family, friends, church and community. Those strong emotional ties of love that bind us mean it is natural for us to want to remain in the world.

The believer will have a passion to serve God in this world, to bear fruit for God's glory. Yet, at the same time, our eternal home is in heaven and that is what we long for. We can be torn between these two places. The apostle Paul wrote to the Philippian church:

> *If I am to go on living in the body, this will mean fruitful labour for me. Yet what shall I choose? I do not know! I am torn between the two: I desire to depart and be with Christ, which is better by far; but it is more necessary for you that I remain in the body. Convinced of this … I will continue with all of you for your progress and joy in the faith.*
>
> (Philippians 1:22-25)

## Prayer for healing

Clearly, it is not wrong to pray for your own physical healing or for the healing of a family member or for the church to pray in this way. Karen and I regularly pray that the treatment that I am on will be effective. We also desire to serve the Lord and see fruitful labour including the 'progress and joy in the faith' of the church (verse 25)—and we regularly pray for that too.

Of course, our Father in heaven knows and cares for all the details of our lives. Scripture calls us to bring our burdens to God (Psalm 55:22). Therefore, it is right to pray for healing as an individual and as a church. Will God always answer that prayer for healing? As with all prayers, God may answer 'yes', 'no' or 'wait'. We may find it hard to comprehend but we do know God's will is for our good and is best. It is important to remember that there is a sense in which God will *always* answer that prayer for complete healing with a 'Yes!', for those who believe. God will answer that prayer in an incredible way when he takes his people to be with Jesus Christ in heaven. That is true, complete and ultimate healing. This is far better than anything in this world.

The prayer that our body will be fully healed will be fully answered, ultimately and perfectly, when we are given a new resurrected body and when we are in heaven for ever.[21] There will be no more cancer in our body, no more sickness, no more tears, no more sorrow, no more heartache and no more death. God may give us a measure of healing on earth—and we praise God for it. But that healing will be imperfect—as one day, sooner or later, we will die. If God was to perfectly heal all the bodies of Christians on earth, then they would never go to heaven!

It is important to remember that everyone who the Lord Jesus 'healed' during his three years of ministry on earth later took sick and died. Therefore, it is only in heaven that we will never be sick and we will never die. We must understand that there is a *future* aspect to our salvation which is the redemption of our body, when we receive a new glorified body at the resurrection on the last day.

However, here on earth our bodies outwardly waste away in this world of death and decay.

> *Therefore we do not lose heart. Though outwardly we are wasting away, yet inwardly we are being renewed day by day. For our light and momentary troubles are achieving for us an eternal glory that far outweighs them all. So we fix our eyes not on what is seen, but on what is unseen, since what is seen is temporary, but what is unseen is eternal.*
> (2 Corinthians 4:16-18)

When viewed in the light of eternity, all our troubles in this decaying world are temporary and fleeting. Therefore, physical healing, if we receive it, is only temporary. This world is fleeting and passing away. James says:

> *What is your life? You are a mist that appears for a little while and then vanishes.* (James 4:14)

I looked out of the kitchen window of my home in Ahoghill some years ago and all I could see was a white haze, because the morning mist had come down. I could not see the garden, or the field beyond that and the road beyond that. In the afternoon, I looked out of the same kitchen window and I could clearly see the garden, the field and the road. The morning mist was gone a few hours after it first appeared. In comparison to eternity, our life in this world is like a morning mist. We are only here in the world for a short time.

## This brief life

On one occasion, I conducted the funeral of a lady who died in her nineties. But even the longest life in this world is so brief in the light of eternity. Eternity lasts forever. Heaven lasts forever. Therefore, let us live in the light of eternity and fix our eyes on the eternal hope of being with Christ in heaven which is far better. Let us rejoice and celebrate this sure and certain hope we have in Jesus Christ and live daily for God's glory.

However, when we are going through acute suffering, we often cannot see the hand of God or the purpose of God. We do not have a Biblical perspective. The day I was diagnosed with incurable, in-operable cancer on the 6 November 2017, my mind was in a spin. I woke up during that night sorely afraid and felt that God had abandoned me. I felt he had forsaken me. I was so afraid of death. When I was in the midst of the fierce storm, nothing seemed to make sense and I was confused. I was overwhelmed and completely disorientated. Yet now, looking back, God was never absent from me or ever abandoned me or forsook me.

*God has said:*
*'Never will I leave you; never will I forsake you.'*
*So we say with confidence,*
*'The Lord is my helper: I will not be afraid.'*

(Hebrews 13:5-6)

Even when I was in that dark place the Lord was my helper and was near me, even when my feelings were mixed up. God brought me through and sustained me. I praise God that he is the Father of compassion and the God of all comfort (2 Corinthians 1:3). He does not treat us as our sins deserve but, as far as the east is from the west, he removes our transgressions from us (Psalm 103:10-11).

## Unexpected blessings

I am so thankful to God for the measure of earthly healing the Lord has given me. I never expected to be alive two years and six months after my diagnosis for incurable cancer. We should never doubt the power of Almighty God who is able to do immeasurably more than all we ask or imagine. 'Understanding aright, the gracious power of God results in a faith that expects God to minister to us in our time of need.'[22] God loves us and sustains us in our time of need. We are able to face death and make preparations to do so. I am not afraid of dying. Why not? Let me share my story and tell you why.

When I was twenty-two years of age, I had given up on church and any form of religion. I was simply wanting to enjoy myself in life. Then I almost had a serious car accident on the way to Portrush. A few days later, I woke up in the morning, struggling to breathe, and I was rushed into the Belfast City Hospital. The doctor diagnosed a panic attack or anxiety attack and I was admitted to the Belfast City Hospital. I was lying in a bed in a ward and I asked myself the question, 'If I died today, would I be going to heaven?' I knew I had no chance of going to heaven as I was living merely for myself and was frequently drunk at weekends. Then I wondered, 'If I am not going to heaven, where else do you go?' I thought about hell and I became aware that, because of my sin, hell was my destination. I became very afraid of dying because I knew I was unprepared to meet a holy God as my judge. Hebrews 9:27 says, 'man is destined to die once, and after that to face judgement.'

Later that day, I was discharged from the hospital and I decided I wanted to travel home to Ahoghill for comfort from my parents. As I was driving along the motorway out of Belfast, I knew my life was in a mess and I wondered how God would ever forgive someone like me. Then I remembered what a Sunday teacher had told me and I prayed, 'Come into my life, Lord Jesus. Come in today, Come in to stay. Come into my life, Lord Jesus'.

Tears rolled down my cheeks and I felt broken before God. The Lord Jesus came into my life by the Spirit and I was saved by God's grace. I also became aware for the first time that the devil had a grip on my life and the Lord Jesus had come to deliver me and set me free (1 John 3:8). Later on that day, I talked with the minister of my home congregation, Dr Harry Uprichard. He explained the importance of repentance and turning away from sin in sorrow and hatred of it. He also explained the significance of the cross at Calvary. I had never understood how someone's death nearly 2,000 years ago could have an impact in my life today. But as the minister explained so clearly how much God loved me and that Jesus Christ had died in my place, taking the penalty and punishment that my sins deserved, I understood it for the first time. I was amazed at what the Lord had done for a sinner like me. I was overwhelmed. So, in response, I gave my life to Jesus, asking him to be my Saviour and Lord. Jesus died to bring me forgiveness from my sins and he rose again from the dead to give me hope beyond the grave.

## A new beginning

That day marked a new beginning in my life because, for the first time in my life, I discovered the joy of sins forgiven and peace with God. I was no longer afraid of death because now I had the assurance I was going to heaven. Since that day over thirty-four years ago, I have continued to have that assurance of going to heaven. Acts 2:21 says that, 'everyone who calls on the name of the Lord will be saved.'

> *It is no secret what the Lord can do,*
> *What he has done for others,*
> *He can do for you.*[23]

I have made preparations for my funeral service. I am able to 'look death in the eye' and say that because Jesus Christ has conquered death, then so will I.[24] I have chosen the hymns, the Bible reading, the person who will sing and the person to preach. I have chosen the plot of ground in Clough Presbyterian Church graveyard where my body will be buried. I have also made a will. Making a will is good to do to prevent disappointment, family squabbles and potential division in the future. Careful and wise planning is essential.

I am thankful to God and have a great debt of gratitude I owe to the National Health Service in Northern Ireland. I have visited Accident and Emergency units at Daisy Hill Hospital in Newry and the Royal Victoria Hospital in Belfast. I have been an in-patient at the Daisy Hill Hospital in Newry, Craigavon Area Hospital, and Downe Hospital in Downpatrick. I am now under the care of the Oncology Department at the Bridgewater Suite at the Belfast City Hospital. I have great admiration and deep appreciation for the dedication and commitment of the whole team of health care professionals, consultants, doctors, nurses, receptionists, auxiliary staff, and so on. Their skill, care and expertise has been a great blessing to me. Many have gone the extra mile to show kindness to me when I have been in a vulnerable and weak position. I am also thankful to God for the medical advances that have taken place and the new drugs that are increasingly available in the battle against cancer. God is able to bring recovery to someone who is ill by means of consultants, medical treatments and procedures. At the same time, God is able to work apart from the medical profession if he so chooses. Prayer always plays an important part in what God does in this world.

In conclusion, let us never forget that it is not the *quantity* of our days that matters, but the *quality* of our service for the Lord that counts. Are we living each day to please the Lord? Jim Elliot was born in 1927 in Portland, Oregon, in USA. He trusted in the Lord Jesus as his Saviour when he was just six years old. He graduated from Wheaton College at the age of twenty-one. His heart was in mission, so he travelled to Ecuador in 1952 with the purpose of evangelising Ecuador's Huaorani Indians. In 1953, he married Elisabeth Howard, who was a graduate of Wheaton College and a missionary. Their only child, Valerie, was born in 1955. In 1958, Jim and four other missionaries were speared to death at the Curaray River by those they had come to share the gospel with. Jim died at the age of only twenty-eight. He is now 'away from the body and at home with the Lord' (2 Corinthians 5:8). He has gone to his permanent home in heaven, to be with the Lord. On the 28 October 1949, when he was twenty-two years of age, he wrote the following in his journal:

> *He is no fool who gives what he cannot keep to gain that which he cannot lose.*[25]

## Chapter 10

# Finding wisdom during Covid-19

The name 'coronavirus' is derived from the Latin word *corona* which means crown or wreath. This name refers to the characteristic appearance of the virus by electron microscopy which has a series of spikes on the surface which resembles a crown. Coronavirus disease or Covid-19 is an infectious disease which has grown very rapidly in our world. It was discovered for the first time in Wuhan in China in December 2019. Since then it has spread to 187 countries with over 4 million cases being diagnosed and 284,000 deaths as of 11 May 2020.

In order to prevent the virus from overwhelming the National Health Service and in order to save lives, the United Kingdom has gone into lockdown. The message has been 'Stay at home, save lives'. Social distancing measures have been put in place in order to keep people at least two metres apart. The washing of hands many times a day has become the new norm. As of the 11 May 2020, 223,060 people in the UK have tested positive for the virus and as of 10 May 2020, 32,065 have died. Each person's death is a tragedy.

I remember the leadership in our churches coming together on 17 March 2020 and agreeing to keep all our activities going. Then, less than a week later, we decided to close everything in the church. It felt like a huge tidal wave suddenly striking our church and our country. Later, on 1 April, I received a letter from the Oncology Department asking me to shield from others. I was told not to leave the house for twelve weeks, apart from attending medical appointments.

At times, I felt anxious—certainly in the early days of the virus. If I coughed a few times or I had a sore throat or sore head, I wondered to myself whether I had got the virus. There were times when we had the news on television and I found it was too much to listen to it. We found that the bad news wasn't good for our anxiety levels so we reduced the amount of television we watched and decided to take a break from it completely on a Sunday. How should we respond to this time of crisis in our nation?

## Responding to the crisis

First, we need to lament the terrible suffering and cruel effects of this virus on our world. When we hear of the suffering of families who cannot even see a precious member of their family at the end of their lives, it compounds the pain and heartache. Neither is there a wake or gathering for others to express their sympathy or a service of thanksgiving for their loved one in the church. People are robbed of that support, just when they need it the most. People are not even able to visit members of their families. The virus has resulted in a health crisis, a social crisis, an economic crisis and an educational crisis. People may ask: is there anyone who understands or is able to help us in the dark times of life?

In the Bible, the book of Psalms in the Old Testament is a favourite portion for so many readers, including myself. The psalms cover a wide spectrum of emotions. Some of the 150 psalms are known as of psalms of lament, where moments of great anguish and raw emotion are shared. The psalmist brings his questions to God in Psalm 13:1-2 and Psalm 22:1. The psalmist is open and honest with God. As Todd Billings says, 'In the moments of darkest anguish, the psalmist shows us that God accepts our rawest lament.[26]'

The laments show doubt, anger, pain, confusion, frustration, grief and sadness being expressed in the context of a personal relationship with God. We should never underestimate the sorrows we may face in life—yet we should also never underestimate the love, acceptance and peace we are able to receive from God. It should be noted that in almost all of these types of psalms there is also a note of praise to God. That attitude of gratitude to and worship of God is how we should strive to live each day. Psalm 88 is the exception as there are no specific words of praise. Psalm 88 ends with the words, 'darkness is my closest friend.' Surely this a reminder to us that there may be times in life when we are in the depths of despair and all we are able to do is to pour out our heart to God and wait upon the Lord. At a later date and time, words of praise will come to us. Perhaps these psalms of lament should be read and spoken more often in our churches. Certainly in our pastoral care they are very instructive.

## Weeping at death

In the New Testament, we see Jesus' response to the weeping of Mary and the people after the death of Lazarus. In John 11:35, we read that Jesus wept. Jesus did not weep because Lazarus was dead—we know that because he was coming to raise him from the dead. Jesus was deeply moved not only because of his empathy with Mary but also anger at 'the sin, sickness and death in this fallen world that wrecks so much havoc and generates so much sorrow'.[27] The sufferings of Jesus as the suffering servant are prophesied in Isaiah 53. In Isaiah 53:3, he is described 'a man of suffering, and familiar with pain.'

In the well-known hymn, Jesus is described as a 'man of sorrows'. It is clear that no one ever suffered as much as the Lord Jesus when he experienced the suffering of the cross. He cried out in anguish, 'My God, my God, why have you forsaken me?' (Psalm 22:1, Matthew 27:46). Jesus died as our substitute when he took the condemnation and wrath of God in our place. Jesus was innocent and he took the place of the guilty so that he could bring us to God. The essential point of the Christian faith is that we come to a God who was fully human: he fully understands us in every way and has experienced all the kinds of trials we experience in life. Hebrews 4:15 says, 'For we do not have a high priest who is unable to empathise with our weaknesses, but we have one who has been tempted in every way, just as we have—yet he did not sin.' God has compassion on us. One day in the future, when Jesus Christ brings his people to their eternal home, God's people will leave all their burdens behind them and all their suffering will be over for ever. Revelation 7:17 says, 'God will wipe away every tear from their eyes.' We will then spend eternity forever in the glory of heaven.

## Something is wrong

A second thing we need to understand when we see the cruel effects of this virus—and, indeed, any disaster or tragedy—is that it is a reminder that there is something terribly wrong with this world. The Bible teaches us that when God made the world, it was a perfect place. In the garden of Eden, God enjoyed perfect fellowship and harmony with Adam and Eve. There was perfect harmony between man and the animals as well as the creation itself. However, when Adam and Eve listened to the lies of the devil and disobeyed God by eating of the fruit of the tree of knowledge of good and evil in Genesis 3, spiritual death came into the world. Adam and Eve's relationship with God was fractured and broken, and they were then cast out of the Garden of Eden. In Genesis 3:19, we read about what would happen Adam and Eve, 'you return to the ground'. Physical death came to Adam and Eve and also came into the world. Death, decay and sickness became part of the world which are all the terrible consequences of sin. Ultimately, these are judgements by God on man because of their rebellion. The coronavirus is a reminder to us that all is not well in this world between God and man. It is man's rebellion and sin that has alienated God and erected a barrier between man and God. Yet God in his great mercy has sent his only Son to bring redemption through the death of Jesus on the cross on our behalf so that the barrier would be removed. Jesus rose from the dead to give us hope beyond the grave. One day, when Jesus returns, he will usher in a new heavens and new earth, the home of righteousness (2 Peter 3:13). Therefore, we are able to have hope in this world only through faith in the Lord Jesus Christ. In a blog post on The Gospel Coalition website, Kevin DeYoung said, 'The coronavirus is a natural evil, under God's providential control to be sure, but whose existence is the result of original sin. The root of all human pain and suffering in the world is the rebellion of our first parents—a rebellion that Christ conquered on the cross and will one day wipe away, along with all its sad and sinister effects.'[28]

## Under control

Thirdly, the coronavirus is not simply a mistake of man, nor is it bad luck that it occurred, nor is it an accident of nature. God is sovereign and the virus is 'under God's providential control'.[29] Therefore, God is able to use this virus to speak to our entire world. C. S. Lewis said this: 'Pain insists on being attended to. God whispers to us in our pleasures, speaks in our conscience, but shouts in our pains: it is his megaphone to rouse a deaf world.'[30] So many in our world have been living for pleasure and having a good time. They have been having a party in many different ways—but now the party is over. Like the account of Belshazzar in the book of Daniel, the writing is on the wall because 'you did not honour the God who holds in his hand your life and all your ways' (Daniel 5:23). The king's days were numbered. The writing was on the wall. Death and judgement were coming.

The writing is on the wall today! Therefore, people must repent of their rebellious ways and turn back to God. God is shouting loudly, and his megaphone has been turned up to full at this time of the virus to rouse people from their spiritual slumber to seek mercy from God before it is too late.

God is not only speaking to the world at this time—he is also speaking to the church, and that includes me. God is using the virus to rouse a deaf church. I wonder, have we been too busy serving the Lord, like the church in Ephesus in Revelation 2:1-7, but have no time for the Lord himself. We hurry through our quiet times to get on with the 'real work', yet our personal relationship with the Lord is neglected and peripheral. We have forsaken our first love. We need to remember the height from which we have fallen and repent.

> *Visit us, Lord, with revival:*
> *Stricken with coldness and death.*
> *Where is our hope of survival,*
> *Save in Thy life-giving breath?* [31]

We desperately need revival, as individuals and as a church, as the old hymn says.

I wonder, have we been so comfortable, materialistic and affluent in the church in the West that we need to re-examine our priorities? Are we like the church at Laodicea in Revelation 3 that is merely lukewarm? Are our priorities in line with the teaching of the Word of God? Do we care for the poor, the persecuted and the needy in other lands or are we too inward looking? Do we need to humble ourselves, pray and seek God's face? Do we need to turn from our wicked ways, so that God will hear us from heaven, forgive our sin and bring healing to our land (2 Chronicles 7:14)? This is a massive challenge to me, as well as each one of us.

## A time of opportunity

Fourthly, the trials associated with the coronavirus provide a wonderful opportunity for the Christian for spiritual growth. James 1:2-4 says,

> *Consider it pure joy, my brothers and sisters, whenever you face trials of many kinds, because you know that the testing of your faith produces perseverance. Let perseverance finish its work so that you may be mature and complete, not lacking anything.*

When James mentions joy in trial, it seems to make no sense at all. This seems so hard to believe and understand. It seems absurd and crazy. The joy is not found in the trial itself but in how God is able to use the trial and work through it to build us up spiritually and strengthen our faith. Instead of complaining and grumbling in our struggles and difficulties, which is natural, we should understand that trials can bring benefit and blessing to our lives. Trials provide an opportunity for us to grow. We need a Biblical and eternal perspective on our trials. Without trials we would be weak, immature and deficient in faith.

## Rejoicing in trials

Some years ago, I flew as a passenger in a Short 360 aircraft between Newcastle and George Best Belfast City airport. At various times, there was a significant amount of turbulence on that journey home. The plane was buffeted by the strong headwinds that were against it. The quality and strength of the metal used in the construction of that aircraft would have been severely tested in the laboratory before it would have been safely and securely used in the operation of the aircraft. So too, the Christian's faith needs to be severely tested by the strong headwinds and storms of life in order to show it is secure, real and not false. It is possible to rejoice in trials knowing the Lord is with us in them and that he loves us. The trial is not meaningless but God has ultimately designed and permitted the trial, with good purposes in mind. It is sometimes said that even when we are not able to trace God's hand, we are still able to trust God's heart.[32] James provides a wonderful promise to those who persevere and stand the test: they will receive the crown of life (James 1:12). James also warns us that in time of trial, there is real temptation to sin which we must resist.

Romans 8 reminds us that in all things, God is working for our good (verse 28)—and that includes the good of the church which is so precious to Christ. God is working for our good even during the pandemic. It is interesting to note that this well-known verse is written in the context of the reality of 'present sufferings' in this world (verse 18). Creation itself was 'subjected to frustration' by God and is in bondage to decay. This refers to the consequences of the Fall, our inward groaning (verse 23), our questioning, confusion and 'weakness' as 'we do not know what we ought to pray' (verse 26). God is therefore working for our good even in the times of suffering, when everything appears to be against us.

Trials such as Covid-19—and many other trials too—are an inevitable part of the fallen and decaying world in which we live but God is able to use them to develop our Christian character, and also use us as his witnesses through them. So we are enabled by God's Spirit to grow—in love for others, in boldness when we share our faith, and in usefulness. Recently, I changed my mobile phone and I needed some technical support. I was talking to an adviser on the telephone and I asked him where he came from. To my great surprise, he told me that he came from Cairo where the call centre was situated and that he was a student. I asked him if he had read the Bible and he replied that he had read parts of it. I shared that I had incurable cancer and I was not afraid of death because Jesus Christ had saved me by his grace. He said he had not heard that message before. He then explained it was the best call he had taken in his life. Surely God had opened a door for the gospel.

## Such a time as this

During the pandemic, our churches in Clough and Seaforde have been active on Facebook, on our church website and our YouTube channel to proclaim the gospel and the unsearchable riches that are found in Christ. Like so many evangelical churches, many more people are listening and watching than ever before. The church buildings may be empty but so is the grave of our Saviour who has sent the Holy Spirit to equip us for 'such a time as this'. Mordecai asks Queen Esther to help the Jews at a crucial time and said, 'who knows but that you have come to your royal position for such a time as this?' (Esther 4:14). God has providentially brought us to our positions and our circumstances in life for such a crucial time as this in our nation for his purposes. Let us seize the day. Let us act with vision, faith and self-denying love. Let us not hoard but give generously. Let us not be anxious but pray and rejoice. There is no telling how the Lord will use us who belong to his church, for his glory.

# Chapter 11

# Finding a future home?

***Karen writes:***

As I have already shared, at times, my mind wanders. Sometimes this is not good, as all sorts of notions and thought processes go through my head. In my mind, I take myself to a place where Adrian is no longer with me and I contemplate how I will navigate life without him. It breaks my heart to think of the possibility of being separated from him, and leaving my home that the church has provided for us both. But God is already there and he knows the path that I take. How lovely is Job 23:10, 'He knows the way that I take, when he has tested me, I will come forth as gold'. I do not allow my mind to dwell on the negative, it's not healthy for me in any way, so I have to keep my eyes firmly on the Lord.

## Fighting for life

We are fully aware that Adrian's diagnosis, medically speaking, is indeed bleak so I am also aware of the humanness of our situation. But I can also say confidently that my faith, trust and dependence is in God. I believe that the Lord can heal and restore Adrian—and when you are in the place that we are presently in, every cell in your body wants to fight for life. That is a natural instinct on our part. I have also learned that Adrian does not belong to me. It is easy to have this notion that our spouse is ours, but he is not mine. He belongs to the Lord Jesus, who paid the highest cost possible to redeem Adrian back to himself, through his shed blood at Calvary. I also know that my identity is in Christ Jesus and, no matter what my status is or will be in the future, my life is indeed secure and hidden in him.

I encourage you to read Isaiah 54. I love these verses, especially verse five:

> *For your Maker is your husband –*
> *the Lord Almighty is his name –*
> *the Holy One of Israel is your Redeemer,*
> *he is called the God of all the earth.*

Does that not excite you? It amazes me. To think that the single woman craving a husband of her own, the grieving widow broken with grief and loneliness, the divorced woman crushed by heartache, rejection and disappointment all have a 'husband' who will never leave, hurt, reject or abandon them. This husband is Jesus Christ himself, the lover of our souls. The mountains may shake,

> *'yet my unfailing love for you will not be shaken, nor my covenant of peace be removed' says the Lord, who has compassion on you.* (Isaiah 54:10)

Cancer has certainly shaken us as a couple and there are many reasons why as Christians we can be shaken in our lives. Of course, it doesn't have to be cancer, like it is for Adrian and me. Whatever it is, there is his 'covenant of peace' to sustain and carry us through the hardest of times.

## Preparing a home

And so, as I conclude, the Lord, my 'husband'—and for you who know and love him, *our* husband—is away preparing the most wonderful home for his bride. The Bible tells us that no eye has seen, no ear has heard, and no human mind has conceived the things God has prepared for those who love him (1 Corinthians 2:9). He first prepared a place when he died on the cross at Calvary, rose from the grave, then ascended to Heaven were he resides, reigning in power and majesty. He is preparing a heavenly, eternal home for his bride, the church. He is coming back again, to take us to be with him, so we will be forever with our heavenly bridegroom. There won't be any more cancer there, or anything else that causes pain or heartache to those who love him. Ultimately, my future home is with my heavenly husband, the Lord Jesus himself. Adrian will be there too and all the redeemed from the beginning of time; but Jesus Christ will be the focus and centre of our praise, worship and adoration for all of eternity.

Our dear friend, Gary McDowell, who is also a colleague of Adrian's in the ministry, has written the following song called, 'No Eye Has Seen' for the album 'Facing Cancer: Standing Tall'. Gary and his daughter, Debs, sing the song together. The words are so encouraging and I trust they also encourage and comfort your heart.

*No eye has seen,*
*No ear has heard,*
*No mind has conceived,*
*What God has prepared for those who love Him.*
*For those who love Him, the One,*
*the One who first loved me.*

*I can't imagine what heaven's gonna be,*
*There'll be no tears, there'll be no pain,*
*There'll be no fear when Jesus reigns*
*And we will see Him, the Lamb, upon His throne,*
*And we will worship Jesus,*
*The kingdom of our God will be our home.*

*No eye has seen,*
*No ear has heard,*
*No mind has conceived,*
*What God has prepared for those who love Him,*
*For those who love Him, the One,*
*the One who first loved me.*
*No eye has seen.*[33]

**Adrian writes:**
Seventy years from now, where will Karen and I be? Revelation 7:9-12 provides the answer.

> *After this I looked, and there before me was a great multitude that no one could count, from every nation, tribe, people and language, standing before the throne and before the Lamb. They were wearing white robes and were holding palm branches in their hands. And they cried out in a loud voice:*
>
> *'Salvation belongs to our God,*
> *who sits on the throne,*
> *and to the Lamb.'*
>
> *All the angels were standing around the throne and around the elders and the four living creatures. They fell down on their faces before the throne and worshiped God, saying:*
>
> *'Amen!*
> *Praise and glory*
> *and wisdom and thanks and honour*
> *and power and strength*
> *be to our God for ever and ever.*
> *Amen!'*

Karen and I will be gathered along with a great multitude of people from every nation. People from Australia, China, Nigeria, Uganda, Brazil, Israel, Syria, Italy, Poland, the United Kingdom and the Republic of Ireland. We will be standing before God's throne in heaven. We will be wearing white robes, which symbolises purity and cleansing from all defilement. That cleansing from sin has been accomplished by the Lamb's sacrificial death. We will be holding palm branches, which speaks of a festive occasion and celebration. We will be singing. What will we be singing about? Salvation is found in God alone and his Son, the Lamb of God who died and rose again. We will be joined by the saints and angels in the worship and praise of God.

> *For the Lamb at the centre of the throne will be their shepherd; 'he will lead them to springs of living water.' 'And God will wipe away every tear from their eyes.' (Revelation 7:17)*

Jesus, the divine Shepherd-Lamb, leads his people to abundant life. There will be no more cancer or tears or sorrow or heartache or death. Together, Jesus and his people will enjoy and celebrate who God is and what the Lord Jesus Christ has done for them for ever and ever and ever.

> *When we've been there ten thousand years,*
> *Bright shining as the sun,*
> *We've no less days to sing God's praise*
> *Than when we first begun.*[34]

Appendix

# Some poems and a song

## A cancer poem for the Christian

*This poem is based on the 'What Cancer Cannot Do' poem, author unknown, found in many different places on the internet.*

Cancer appears so very strong—but its power is limited.
Cancer cannot... rob us of our joy
(1 Peter 1:8)
Cancer cannot... squash our peace
(Philippians 4:7)
Cancer cannot... bury our hope
(Hebrews 6:19)
Cancer cannot... quell our love
(Ephesians 1:4-5)
Cancer cannot... extinguish our faith
(Ephesians 2:8)
Cancer cannot... hinder our spiritual growth
(2 Peter 1:3)
Cancer cannot... blot out the memories of family and friends
(Psalm 68:6)
Cancer cannot... destroy God's great salvation
(Revelation 7:9-10)
Cancer cannot... wreck God the Father's plans for our lives
(Psalm 33:11)

Cancer cannot... separate us from Jesus Christ's love
(Romans 8:35-39)
Cancer cannot... remove the Holy Spirit's power
(2 Timothy 1:7)
Cancer cannot... ruin God's purposes for our future
(Romans 8:28-30)
Cancer cannot... defeat the resurrection of the body
(1 Corinthians 15:51-55)
Cancer cannot... take eternal life from us
(John 10:27-28)
Cancer cannot... prevent us going to heaven
(1 Peter 1:3-4)
Cancer cannot... take away our sins, only the Lord Jesus is able
(1 John 1:7)

## My Adrian—a poem by Karen

*My Daddy walked me along the aisle,*
*To meet you there with beaming smile*
*You took my hand, I let go of his,*
*Focused on my bridegroom's eyes.*

*There could have been an empty room,*
*For all that mattered on that moment*
*Was you and I, and the God who planned it.*

*The vows were said,*
*We meant each word,*
*The promises to one another;*
*A covenant to be unbroken,*
*Rings exchanged,*
*God's Word spoken.*

*We started life*
*As new man and wife,*

*A few years in—pretty perfect.*
*Then a pain in the side,*
*We cried and cried,*
*For the cancer so unexpected.*

*The vows are still true,*
*To this day, I love you*
*Yet more through the trials it's deepened.*

*On God's Word we rely,*
*till the day we both die*
*His love even then more steepened.*

*And yet we're standing tall together,*
*Sunshine, rain, whatever the weather*

*Cancer's not our identity,*
*It's Christ in us and Him in me.*

*Sickness, health,*
*Poor or in wealth*
*We're united in life and eternity.*

## Missing You—a poem by Karen

*Clough and Seaforde, we really miss you!*
*Self- isolating, bit less to do.*
*Yet the weeks are passing by;*
*I've laughed and cried and said, 'Oh why?'*
*Been no church for quite a while;*
*We miss you all, each voice, every smile.*

*It's not easy being stuck inside,*
*A deadly virus from whom we must hide;*
*Loneliness, fear, yes; that can be true,*
*Upset, tears—all shed by you.*
*But on God's Word we must abide.*

*Self-isolating? No, he never leaves your side.*

*Each person, family, you all matter.*
*WhatsApp, Facebook, on the phone we natter.*
*God's Word opened more, in our homes each day;*
*Reading, meditating, special times to pray.*

*Church services? Yes, we've missed a few.*
*Buildings closed, an empty pew.*
*Yet Clough and Seaforde, standing strong,*
*God's Word in our hearts; on our lips a song.*
*Weeks or months? I could be wrong;*
*Adrian and I—with you all belong.*

## Facing Cancer: Standing Tall—a song by Gary McDowell

*Facing cancer standing tall.*
*If it were not for the grace of God,*
*I would not stand at all.*
*Facing cancer but I see Jesus.*
*I stand upon this rock and I won't fall.*
*Standing tall.*

*Being confident of this*
*That he who started a good work in you will finish.*
*He is faithful. He is true*
*And the hope you have does not depend on you.*

*Trust in the Lord with all your heart*
*And lean not on your own understanding*
*In all your ways acknowledge Him*
*And He'll direct your path, he'll direct your path.*

*Facing cancer standing tall.*
*If it were not for the grace of God,*
*I would not stand at all.*
*Facing cancer but I see Jesus.*

*I stand upon this rock and I won't fall*
*Standing tall.*

*When you pass through the waters,*
*He will be with you, he will be with you.*
*When you pass through the rivers,*
*You're still in His care, You're still in His care.*
*When you walk through the fire,*
*He won't desert you, he won't desert you.*
*For didn't he promise, didn't he say,*
*Wherever you go He'll be there?*

*Facing cancer standing tall.*
*If it were not for the grace of God,*
*I would not stand at all.*
*Facing cancer but I see Jesus.*
*I'll stand upon this rock and I won't fall.*

*Facing cancer but I'm standing tall.*
*I'm standing tall.*[35]

# Resources

## Videos

A friend, Jonny Sanlon, who is a videographer, has helped us to put our story into a series of five short videos. A number of people have told us that they have found these very helpful. We have also shared our testimonies and given some Bible teaching. Two music videos and two videos about what led Gary McDowell to write the songs are also available. Karen also shows how to make scones, banana bread and ice cream! You can watch them all by visiting:

- Our church website
  https://www.cloughandseaforde.com
- Our church Facebook page
  https://www.Facebook.com/CloughandSeafordePresbyterian
- Our church YouTube channel—Clough and Seaforde
  https://www.youtube.com

## CD

As described in chapter 8, our story is also featured on a CD—'Facing Cancer: My journey to finding joy (in word and song)'. We are so grateful to the fantastic team that made this possible: in particular, Gordy McCracken, Gary McDowell, Hannah McPhillimy, Janet Young, Debs McDowell, Roy Rainey, Mark Rainey and Jonny Sanlon. Special thanks to Andrew Forson for permission to use Castlewellan Castle Christian Conference centre for filming. Available from the bookshops listed below.

## Endnotes


1. John Piper, 'Christ and Cancer', 17 August 1980, https://www.desiringgod.org/messages/christ-and-cancer.
2. Robin Mark, 'Jesus, All for Jesus', https://www.youtube.com/watch?v=H1Wa2msOq9c.
3. Julie Peake, 'Living with Cancer', Presbyterian Church in Ireland, 7 September 2018, https://www.presbyterianireland.org/Blog/September-2018/Living-with-cancer.aspx
4. 'My Heart Is Filled With Thankfulness', words and music by Keith Getty & Stuart Townend, Thankyou Music, 2003.
5. Ian Harbison and Julie Peak, 'The big C… Christ, you and me', https://newhorizon.org.uk/downloads/the-big-c-christ-you-and-me-ian-harbinson-julie-peake/.
6. Travis L. Myers, review of David Powlison's *When Cancer Interrupts*, 3 August 2015, https://www.thegospelcoalition.org/reviews/when-cancer-interrupts/.
7. Kittie Louise Jennett Suffield, 'Little Is Much When God Is In It', 1924.
8. Kevin L. DeYoung, *The Good News We Almost Forgot: Rediscovering the Gospel in a 16th Century Catechism*, Moody Press, 2010.
9. Norman Clayton, 'Now I Belong to Jesus', 1943.
10. Johnson Oatman, 'When upon Life's Billows You are Tempest Tossed', 1987.
11. https://www.facebook.com/CloughandSeafordePresbyterian; https://www.youtube.com/channel/UC304RdF1xYEZ6b_tF7J1vkQ; https://www.cloughandseaforde.com.
12. https://www.facebook.com/kmuganda/ and https://www.instagram.com/kisakyeministries/.
13. William J. and Gloria Gaither, 'God Sent His Son, They Called Him Jesus', 1971.
14. *Westminster Confession of Faith*, 1647.
15. Philip McKelvey, 'Exploring Christian Healing', dissertation for Master of Theology submitted to Faculty of Humanities Institute of Theology, Queens University, September 2005.
16. 'Behold Our God', music and words by Jonathan Baird, Meghan Baird, Ryan Baird, Stephen Altrogge, Sovereign Grace Worship, 2011. Scripture references: Isaiah 25:9, Isaiah 35:4, Isaiah 40:12-17, Psalms 46:6-10.
17. Charles Spurgeon, *Sovereign Grace and Man's Responsibility*, 1 August 1858, https://www.spurgeon.org/resource-library/sermons/sovereign-grace-and-mans-responsibility#flipbook/.
18. Joseph Milicott Scriven, 'What A Friend We Have in Jesus', 1855.
19. McKelvey, 'Exploring Christian Healing'.
20. Myers, review of *When Cancer Interrupts*.
21. Bryan Chappel and Al Mohler, 'Why Doesn't God Always Heal?', 27 January 2020, https://www.thegospelcoalition.org/podcasts/q-a-podcast/why-doesnt-god-always-heal/.
22. McKelvey, 'Exploring Christian Healing'.

23. Stuart Hamblen, 'It Is No Secret', 1950.
24. Myers, review of *When Cancer Interrupts*.
25. Elisabeth Elliot (ed.), *The Journals of Jim Elliot*, Revell, 2002.
26. J. Todd Billings, 'God is Bigger than my Cancer: Learning Joy in the Darkness', 9 May 2015, https://www.desiringgod.org/articles/god-is-bigger-than-my-cancer.
27. D.A. Carson (ed.), *NIV Zondervan Study Bible*, p. 2176.
28. Kevin DeYoung, 'The Coronavirus is a Result of the Fall', 18 March 2020, https://www.thegospelcoalition.org/blogs/kevin-deyoung/the-coronavirus-is-a-result-of-the-fall/.
29. DeYoung, 'The Coronavirus is a Result of the Fall'.
30. C.S. Lewis, *The Problem of Pain*, Centenary Press, 1940.
31. Horace E. Govan (1866-1932), 'Visit Us, Lord, with Revival'.
32. Charles Spurgeon didn't use these exact words but the original idea probably comes from his sermon, 'A Happy Christian', no. 736.
33. 'No Eye Has Seen', words and music by Gary McDowell, performed by Debs and Gary McDowell, film and production by JS Media, 22 March 2020, https://www.youtube.com/watch?v=VF5NQSp7_T0.
34. John Newton, 'Amazing Grace', 1779.
35. 'Facing Cancer: Standing Tall', words and music by Gary McDowell, performed by Debs and Gary McDowell, film and production by JS Media, 15 March 2020, https://www.youtube.com/watch?v=xTHwyE6bqTg.

## Acknowledgements and thanks

Karen and I want to express our heartfelt appreciation to the many who have prayed for us, from a wide spectrum of evangelical churches.

We are so thankful to Rev Dr Sid Garland for guiding us along the process of producing a book. He has continued to be a tremendous mentor and has given us great advice to enable this second book to be written and printed. I greatly appreciate the friendship I have enjoyed with Rev Dr Paul Bailie over the years and we are grateful for the Foreword he has written for our book.

We want to express our deep gratitude to Mary Davis for the godly way that she has helped to produce our manuscript. Mary's tremendous skill, expertise and assistance was invaluable in bringing the second manuscript to completion. We greatly appreciate Tim Thornborough for his wisdom in guiding us through the process from the completion of the manuscript to the printing of another book.

We are so thankful to our friend and videographer Jonny Sanlon for the amazing videos (including music videos) that he has produced on our behalf. We also want to thank him for his help in the production of the photographs for the book.

We are so grateful to Rev Gary McDowell for permission to include the two songs he has written.

*Also by Adrian Adger*

*Avalable from all bookshops listed on the back page*

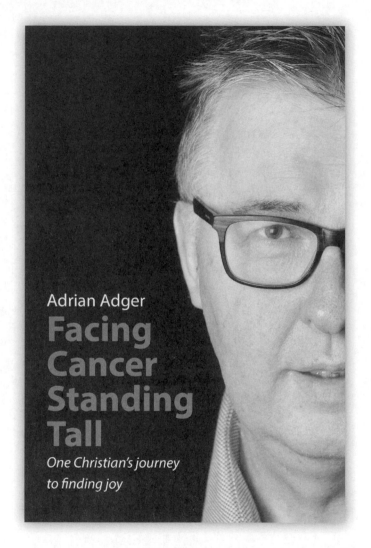

## Copies of this book are available from:

**All Faith Mission** bookshops
in Northern Ireland
www.faithmission.org

**Belfast City Mission**
5th Floor, Glengall Exchange
3 Glengall Street
Belfast BT12 5AB
Tel 028 9032 0557

**Covenanter Bookshop**
www.covenanterbooks.com
37 Knockbracken Road
Carryduff, Belfast BT8 6SE
Tel 028 9081 4110

**Evangelical Bookshop**
15 College Square East
Belfast BT1 6DD
Tel 028 9032 0529

**Mission Africa**
14 Glencregagh Court
Belfast BT6 OPA
Tel 028 9040 2850

**Ards Evangelical Bookshop**
48 Frances Street
Newtownards BT23 7DN
Tel 028 9181 7530

**Beulah Bookshop**
25 Central Promenade
Newcastle, BT33 0AA
Tel 028 4372 2629

**The Secret Place**
18 Rashee Road
Ballyclare BT39 9HJ
Tel 028 9335 2170

**The Burning Bush: Christian Book Centre**
62 Scotch Street
Dungannon BT70 1BJ
Tel 028 8772 6027

**European Mission Fellowship**
23 Millgrange, Ballymoney
County Antrim BT53 7QB
Tel 028 2766 4214

**The Book Well**
27 Belmont Road
Belfast BT4 2AA
Tel 075 8114 3596

**Real Life**
8 Dublin Road, Enniskillen
County Fermanagh BT74 6HH
Tel 028 6632 2400

**Cavan Christian Bookshop**
22a Bridge Street
Cavan, County Cavan
Tel 00 353 4943 61418

*also available on* Amazon.